AF775259

Breast Reconstruction - Conceptual Evolution

Edited by Yueh-Bih Tang

Published in London, United Kingdom

Breast Reconstruction - Conceptual Evolution
http://dx.doi.org/10.5772/intechopen.108086
Edited by Yueh-Bih Tang

Contributors
Angelo Cuzalina, Annabelle Xiao Yan Tan, Dhanushya Gohil, E.V. Vitalievich Shivilov, Emily Louise Hopwood, Ernesto A. Moretti, Evania Lok, Fiona Jane Tsang-Wright, Gurami Elgudzhaevich Kvetenadze, Haruyuki Takata, Hugo St. Hilaire, I.E. Khatkov, K.A. Anichkina, K.S. Arslanov, Karinn Chambers, L.G. Zhukova, Michael Borrero, Márcia Balbina Lorenzo Hoyos, Naoki Watanabe, Pan Dai, Pasquale G. Tolomeo, Raj Manas, Robert Allen, Sally Ng, Sena Hori, Shoko Otsuka, Takeshi Yuasa, Tammy Walker-Smith, Victoria A. Mañón, Xu Hua, Xu Yuanbing

© The Editor(s) and the Author(s) 2024

The rights of the editor(s) and the author(s) have been asserted in accordance with the Copyright, Designs and Patents Act 1988. All rights to the book as a whole are reserved by INTECHOPEN LIMITED. The book as a whole (compilation) cannot be reproduced, distributed or used for commercial or non-commercial purposes without INTECHOPEN LIMITED's written permission. Enquiries concerning the use of the book should be directed to INTECHOPEN LIMITED rights and permissions department (permissions@intechopen.com).

Violations are liable to prosecution under the governing Copyright Law.

Individual chapters of this publication are distributed under the terms of the Creative Commons Attribution 3.0 Unported License which permits commercial use, distribution and reproduction of the individual chapters, provided the original author(s) and source publication are appropriately acknowledged. If so indicated, certain images may not be included under the Creative Commons license. In such cases users will need to obtain permission from the license holder to reproduce the material. More details and guidelines concerning content reuse and adaptation can be found at http://www.intechopen.com/copyright-policy.html.

Notice

Statements and opinions expressed in the chapters are these of the individual contributors and not necessarily those of the editors or publisher. No responsibility is accepted for the accuracy of information contained in the published chapters. The publisher assumes no responsibility for any damage or injury to persons or property arising out of the use of any materials, instructions, methods or ideas contained in the book.

First published in London, United Kingdom, 2024 by IntechOpen
IntechOpen is the global imprint of INTECHOPEN LIMITED, registered in England and Wales, registration number: 11086078, 167-169 Great Portland Street, London, W1W 5PF, United Kingdom

British Library Cataloguing-in-Publication Data
A catalogue record for this book is available from the British Library

Additional hard and PDF copies can be obtained from orders@intechopen.com

Breast Reconstruction - Conceptual Evolution
Edited by Yueh-Bih Tang
p. cm.
Print ISBN 978-1-83768-280-5
Online ISBN 978-1-83768-281-2
eBook (PDF) ISBN 978-1-83768-282-9

We are IntechOpen, the world's leading publisher of Open Access books

Built by scientists, for scientists

7,000+
Open access books available

188,000+
International authors and editors

205M+
Downloads

156
Countries delivered to

Our authors are among the
Top 1%
most cited scientists

12.2%
Contributors from top 500 universities

WEB OF SCIENCE™

Selection of our books indexed in the Book Citation Index
in Web of Science™ Core Collection (BKCI)

Interested in publishing with us?
Contact book.department@intechopen.com

Numbers displayed above are based on latest data collected.
For more information visit www.intechopen.com

For EU product safety concerns:
IN TECH d.o.o., Prolaz Marije Krucifikse Kozulić 3, 51000 Rijeka, Croatia, info@intechopen.com or visit our website at intechopen.com.

Meet the editor

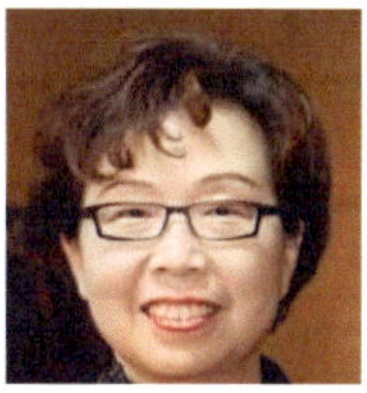

Yueh-Bih Tang is a professor of plastic surgery at the National Taiwan University Hospital, Taipei, Taiwan, and is currently a consulting plastics surgeon at the Far Eastern Memorial Hospital, Banqiao, New Taipei City. She was also the president of the Taiwan Society of Plastic Surgery as well as the Taiwan Aesthetic Surgery Society. Among her academic achievements, it is relevant to highlight her position as a visiting scholar at the Department of Plastic Surgery, Hospital of the University of Pennsylvania and Children Hospital of Philadelphia, and visiting scholar at St. Vincent's Hospital and Royal Melbourne Hospital, Melbourne, Australia.

Contents

Preface

Breast reconstruction is a common problem for women with breast disease or disorder. Early diagnosis of breast cancer is always important for women of any age. Decreasing the morbidity and mortality rate is of utmost importance.

Nowadays, conservation surgery for breast cancer followed by post-operative radiotherapy, hormonal therapy, targeted therapy, and chemotherapy may help decrease the physical and psychological impact on the afflicted patient.

Restoration of the breast form for the sense of being a woman is always anticipated. Various kinds of reconstruction have been developed for patients to select whatever they need. A strategic approach to achieving a satisfactory outcome without being physically handicapped is encouraged.

The contents of this book include the importance of breast screening with an overview of breast disease, new advances in breast cancer treatment, with current surgical and medical treatments. Contributors of chapters are specialists from countries all over the world. Their endeavors in working on the chapters and sharing their precious experiences are deeply appreciated.

Yueh-Bih Tang
National Taiwan University Hospital,
Taipei, Taiwan

Chapter 1

Breast Health and Preventive Screening

Tammy Walker-Smith

Abstract

Breast health and its importance in every stage of a woman's life is discussed from adolescence, across the life span, and addressing the aging process. The importance of self-breast exams, clinical breast exam, and screening mammograms play an integral part of ensuring early detection of breast cancer. The risk factors, genetic mutations, and how breast cancer is triggered is discussed. The advancements in screening recommendations, genetic testing, and treatments is explored and what innovative approaches are being taken to prevent, treat, and cure breast cancer.

Keywords: mammary glands, mammogram, breast cancer screening, BRCA1 & 2 gene, breast cancer, next-generation sequencing, MammaPrint, adjuvant therapy

1. Introduction

The breasts for male and female are similar through childhood where they both have undeveloped breast tissue. This similarity changes for females between ages 8–10 years of age when the breasts begin to develop prior to menarche (start of menses) and continues through puberty [1]. Menarche usually begins around age 12 when the Tanner stage has reached stage 3 or 4. The breasts begin to respond to hormonal changes of increased estrogen during puberty where other changes become evident as well such as pubic hair and hair growth in the axillary region occurs. The breast development process is one that can be described through tanner stages 1–5 in progression until the female breasts are fully developed and rounded with the nipples protruding (see **Table 1**) [1].

Males have breasts that remain basic in function throughout life that is not as complex as the female breast, nor does it have the capability to produce breast milk to breast feed an infant. The obvious breast differences between the two genders provides a platform for discussing the breast anatomy of the female, the response to hormones, and its function(s) [1].

2. Breast anatomy

The breast is comprised of mammary ducts, lobules, fatty tissue, blood vessels, connective tissue, areola, nipples, and lymph nodes. The picture below provides a visual of what a fully developed breast looks like (**Figure 1**) [4].

Female breast stage	Breast changes
Stage 1	Nipple raised in pre-teen stage
Stage 2	Nipple buds begin to develop/widen more as do the breasts begin to grow slightly raised/mound
Stage 3	Breasts continue to enlarge/grow with more glandular tissue development and is flush with the nipple
Stage 4	Breasts are more rounded into a mound and a secondary areolar mound is present
Stage 5	Maturity of the breast is achieved, often with the areola darker and flush with the breast mound

Table 1.
Tanner stages 1–5: [2].

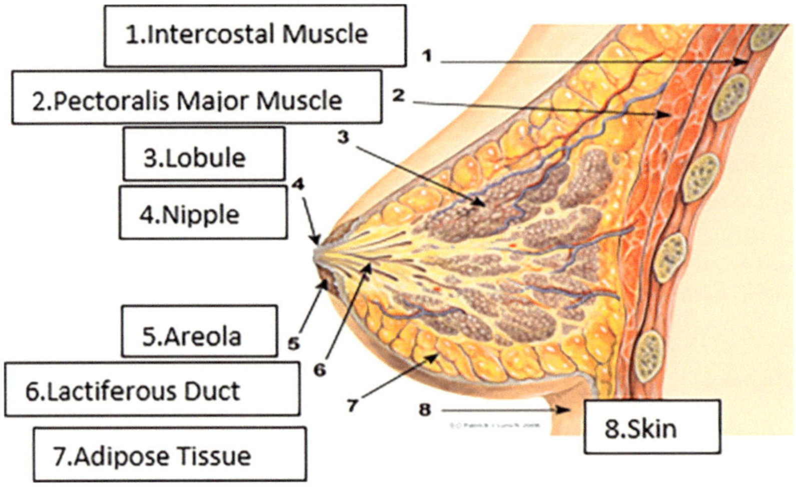

Figure 1.
Breast anatomy Normal Scheme [3].

Breast tissue is derived from lobules and mammary ducts, stroma that is inter and intra lobular in origin, and squamous and epithelial cells. The initial development of lobules (type 1) occurs during puberty. Through the adolescent years, the development of the female breasts continues into early adulthood where type 2 (alveolar maturity) and type-3 lobular mammogenesis (increased breast tissue growth) is triggered by pregnancy [5]. The hormonal changes of higher levels of progesterone and the production of chorionic gonadotropin prepare the breasts to enlarge, lobules to develop further and be able to secrete colostrum and breast milk (lactogenesis) [5].

The breasts' lymph nodes play a significant role in keeping the body healthy by producing lymph fluid and white blood cells called lymphocytes that protect the body from infection and other disease processes. If cancer is present in a specific part of the body, it can shed cancer cells that are either collected through the blood lymph nodes or circulated through the blood vessels. Since the lymph nodes function as a filter, most cancerous cells will remain trapped and not spread to other areas of the body. If cancer cells do escape the lymph node(s), then it can begin to grow in other areas of the body. This process of cancer cells originating in one location and then having a secondary location is known as metastasis (**Figure 2**) [7].

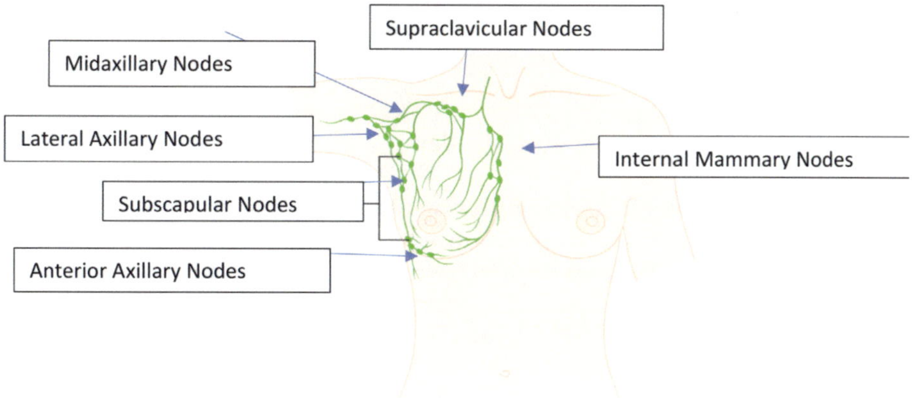

Figure 2.
Lymph nodes of the breast [6].

2.1 Breast feeding

Once the mother delivers her infant, there is a cascade of hormonal processes that occur. The anterior and posterior pituitary gland play a role in hormone stimulation and milk production. Prolactin is regulated by the anterior pituitary and this hormone is released when the infant is breast feeding which triggers the need to produce more milk [5]. Oxytocin, produced in the hypothalamus, is regulated by the posterior pituitary gland for its release. This hormone is released when areolar stimulation from suckling occurs which in turn allows the milk to be released during breast feeding, also known as the "letdown reflex." Oxytocin has additional benefits that relieve stress and assist in the mother's relaxed and calm demeanor [5]. One added benefit of oxytocin is believed to assist in a mother bonding with her infant. A prospective study in Australia conducted over a 15-year period suggests that there is a correlation between non-breast-feeding mothers and those that breast fed for a very brief period and a lack of bonding which may contribute to maternal maltreatment in the form of neglect. This neglect was inversely correlated to the time spent breast feeding, thus the more months an infant was breast fed, the less likely neglect occurred, due to a stronger bonding relationship developed because of oxytocin as mentioned previously. This study's review also found that those who did not breast feed or breast fed for a short period of time had a higher rate of post-partum depression [8].

Milk production or reduction of milk production is regulated by a feedback inhibitor that is based on the intramammary pressure built up from either milk released or milk accumulated and not released. If the pressure is increased from too much milk built up, then milk production will decrease until the excess pressure is relieved and thus a cyclic process occurs to ensure that milk is produced after a feeding to prepare for the next feeding [5].

Breast feeding is a personal choice for many; however, there are multiple benefits to breast feeding an infant. The mother's immunity is passed onto the infant, the composition of the mother's milk provides digesting benefits along with all the nutrients that the infant will need to develop properly. Breast milk helps to protect the infant from obesity and chronic illnesses [5]. There have been several studies that provide data that breast feeding provides long-term benefits to the mother. There are many conditions that are inversely related to breast feeding that lowers the disease process associated with the following conditions: hypertension, hyperlipidemia, diabetes mellites, metabolic syndrome, cardiovascular disease, cerebral vascular accident, breast cancer, ovarian cancer, endometrial cancer, and rheumatoid arthritis [8].

2.2 Mature breast changes aged 40 and older

Aging breasts often begin to change during perimenopause and after achieving menopause when hormone levels, especially estrogen and progesterone, begin to decrease, and the breasts begin to sag and become less dense. This process occurs as women enter their 40s and 50s. In review, the breasts developed during puberty due to an increase in estrogen and progesterone, so it makes sense that the decline in these same hormones will cause the decline in breast tissue density and fullness. Subsequently, breast cancer is also associated with aging and 80% of all new breast cancers are diagnosed when the woman is in her 50s or older [9].

Multiple risk factors correlate to a higher risk of breast cancer with age being the primary risk factor to consider for both men and women [10]. Other risk factors include familial history of breast cancer and/or history of BRCA gene mutation confirmation, a personal history of breast cancer, exposure to high radiation levels, excessive hormone therapy, age of menarche, Ashkenazi Jewish lineage, and age of first delivery [9]. Other relative risk factors include: higher socioeconomic status, never having had children, alcohol use, did not breast feed, reached menopause after age 55, postmenopausal obesity, and pregnancy after age 30 [1]. These risk factors coupled with age related mammary changes make breast tissue more susceptible to tumor-related mutation in conjunction with lower tumor suppressor effectiveness/response, and damage from exposure to environmental components that may also contribute to changes in breast tissue [11].

Changes in the aging breast from exposure to environmental, hereditary, hormonal, and multiple other risk factors provides insight into the alterations in the cellular and genetic expression of "hormone-sensing and secretory-alveolar lineage markers" as well as inflammatory processes that may contribute to genetic expression mutations [11, 12]. When you combine inflammation with declining bodily function, older age, weight gain (harbors estrogen), and macrophage infiltrative processes together, then you have a recipe for a tumor microenvironment (TME). TMEs are comprised of tumor mediators and tumor cells that regulate the proliferation and metastasis of breast cancer, and it is a good indicator of breast cancer prognosis, especially triple negative breast cancer [12]. Macrophage infiltration prompts a domino effect that activates myeloid-epithelial-reproductive tyrosine kinase (MER TK), which in the right microenvironment, promotes the mutated genetic expression instead of repairing the original genetic expression [13]. The negative affect of MER TK activation for aberrant expression includes hindering cell apoptosis and the expedited activation of metastasis that is resistant to cancer treatments [13].

3. Breast cancer screening and recommendations

Breast cancer screening recommendations from the United States Preventive Services Task Force (USPSTF) provide guidance for women aged 40 and over on breast cancer screening frequency. Since 2016, the recommendation has been for women aged 40–49 to speak with their physician and determine whether every other year screening mammograms is appropriate for them. However, the recommendations are currently being updated to suggest that women aged 40–49 begin screening mammograms every other year. It is recommended that women aged 50–74 maintain routine screening mammograms every other year [14]. The American Cancer Society (ACS) has slightly different recommendations with women aged 40–45 choosing to have annual screening mammograms and women aged 45–54 with annual screening mammograms, and women aged 55 and older to have screening mammograms every other year [9]. The American College of Obstetricians and Gynecologists (ACOG) recommends screening mammograms every 1–2 years for women aged 40–75 [9].

The USPTF and the ACS do not recommend clinical breast examinations and/or self-breast examinations; however, ACOG recommends clinical breast examinations every 1–3 years but no self-breast examinations [9]. These recommendations provide guidance, but to give patients the tools to make informed decisions about their healthcare and body is imperative. Teaching your patients and/or significant other how to examine their breasts once a month empowers self-care, self-awareness, and early detection. Why is this important? Abnormalities identified through patients performing breast self-exams account for 40% of all breast cancer diagnosis [15]. When a patient comes into a clinic and states that they have a lump in their breast, the first question that will be asked of the patient encompasses two parts: (1) "How long has this lump been there?" and (2) "How much has it grown since you found it?" If the patient cannot answer either of these two important questions, then there will be great anxiety from the patient as to what is not known and/or what to expect going forward. Being able to answer these questions helps to gauge the aggressiveness of the lump/mass. Once a history and clinical breast exam is conducted, then a diagnostic mammogram or US should be ordered, depending on their age [16].

With the increase in transgender women on the rise, combined with estrogen hormone therapy, and androgen hormone blocking therapies, it is important to mention that breast cancer is increasing among this population. The reasons vary, but could be contributed to: continuous use of exogenous hormone therapies, the patient's inability to feel a lump due to possible breast augmentation, lack of education with the patient on how to do a breast self-examination, lack of knowledge from primary care providers on how to care for transgender patients, and/or a current lack of screening recommendations for this diverse population [10]. This evolving group of patients will need to begin to assume the risk that ciswomen have and begin to think in these terms to assess their genetic risk of breast cancer and screen accordingly [10].

The rate of breast cancer among men is much lower than it is form women, however, there are still similarities in risk factors such as age, familial history of breast cancer or BRCA1 or 2 mutation, obesity, and radiation exposure. Other risk factors that women do not have is as follows: testicular disorders, Klinefelter syndrome, and gynecomastia (enlarged breasts for men) [10]. Men have a rate of breast cancer incidence of 1.2 per 100,000 men and this accounts for only 1% of all breast cancer diagnosis between 2015 and 2019. Unfortunately, with so little known about male breast cancer, the signs are often overlooked until it is diagnosed at a later cancer stage, usually regional or distant, which makes it harder to treat and correlates to a lower survival rate compared to women [10]. Black men have a higher rate of breast cancer overall as well as sub-types compared to other ethnicities [10]. There is still a lot of work to do to inform men about their risk of breast cancer and when to get checked, but with the help of primary care providers, this can be a conversation that occurs during an annual well check visit.

3.1 Breast cancer risk assessment tool

The Breast Cancer Risk Assessment Tool (BCRAT) is a tool that determines the risk one has over a 5-year and lifetime risk based on their individualized risk factors to provide a risk score prediction that is valid among all ethnicities [17]. This tool allows patients to see if they fall within normal risk levels for their age, ethnicity, familial history of breast cancer, BRCA1 & 2 mutation positive status, and other risk factors, or do they have a higher than normal risk prediction that would encourage more frequent and/or earlier screenings coupled with greater patient compliance with completing routine screening mammograms [18]. There are three sections to this questionnaire: patient eligibility, demographics, and patient and family history (see **Figure 3**).

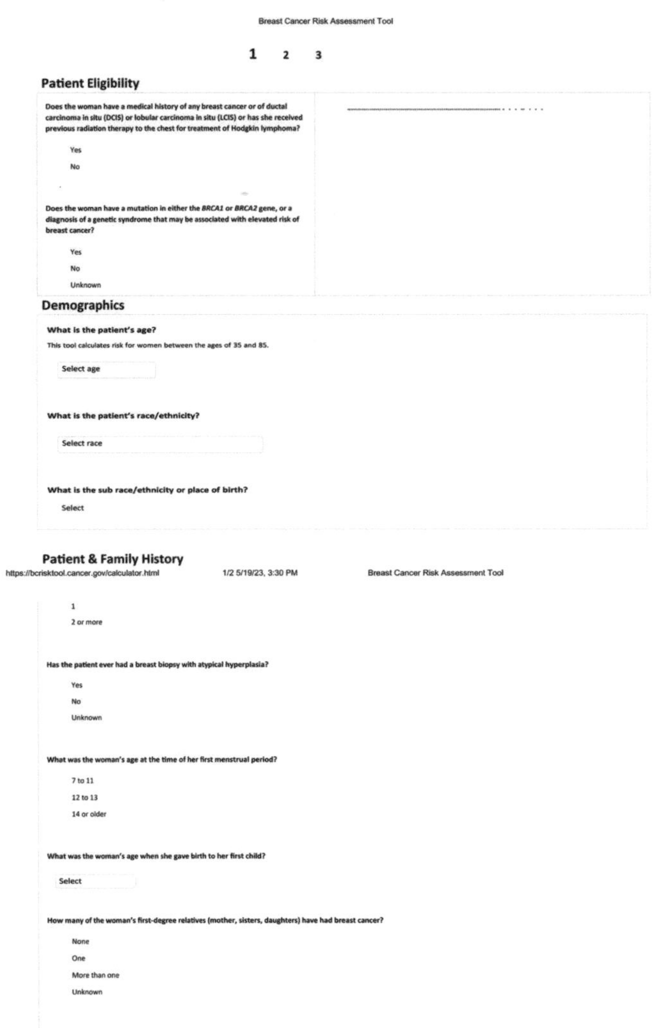
Breast Cancer Risk Assessment Tool

1 2 3

Patient Eligibility

Does the woman have a medical history of any breast cancer or of ductal carcinoma in situ (DCIS) or lobular carcinoma in situ (LCIS) or has she received previous radiation therapy to the chest for treatment of Hodgkin lymphoma?

Yes

No

Does the woman have a mutation in either the *BRCA1* or *BRCA2* gene, or a diagnosis of a genetic syndrome that may be associated with elevated risk of breast cancer?

Yes

No

Unknown

Demographics

What is the patient's age?

This tool calculates risk for women between the ages of 35 and 85.

Select age

What is the patient's race/ethnicity?

Select race

What is the sub race/ethnicity or place of birth?

Select

Patient & Family History

https://bcrisktool.cancer.gov/calculator.html 1/2 5/19/23, 3:30 PM Breast Cancer Risk Assessment Tool

1

2 or more

Has the patient ever had a breast biopsy with atypical hyperplasia?

Yes

No

Unknown

What was the woman's age at the time of her first menstrual period?

7 to 11

12 to 13

14 or older

What was the woman's age when she gave birth to her first child?

Select

How many of the woman's first-degree relatives (mother, sisters, daughters) have had breast cancer?

None

One

More than one

Unknown

https://bcrisktool.cancer.gov/calculator.html

Figure 3.
Breast cancer risk assessment tool [19].

3.2 Genetic counseling and testing

There are two types of genetic mutations that differentiate the origin of the specific type of breast cancer. This will be key in genetic counseling conversations. Germline mutations are inherited because of mutations coded in either the egg and/or sperm cells, such as BRCA1 & 2 mutations that inhibits DNA repairs from occurring naturally. Then there is the somatic mutation which is not inherited and is the direct result of damaged cells with DNA repairs misaligned during restructuring. There is a proportional relationship between somatic mutations and replication accelerated in malignant cancer cells [20]. Also, since BRCA1 & 2 mutations are inherited, patients may find out about their personal risk from other family members and/or simply learn of the higher risk score because of the BCRAT questionnaire and knowledge of known family members having had breast cancer [20]. This crucial information can play an important role in a provider referring the patient to a genetic counselor and having the ability to test for this mutation and take proactive steps in routine screenings instead of waiting and worrying to see if they get breast cancer [21].

Patients with a family history of breast cancer and/or a family member with a positive BRCA1 or 2 gene mutation test will have many questions about their risk and may have scored very high on the BCRAT [19]. The ability to use a risk assessment tool to assist in support and interdisciplinary collaboration between practitioners for patient guidance sets the tone for a patient centered plan of care. Careful planning ensures what the next steps should be: genetic counseling and/or genetic testing, running additional diagnostic testing, and/or scheduling more frequent screenings [22]. Genetic testing is a personal choice and only those with this type of risk should consider having genetic testing as it is very costly and usually not covered by insurance companies. If your patient has a 20% or greater lifetime risk of getting breast cancer, positive for BRCA1 or 2 gene mutation, or has had exposure to chest radiation between the ages of 10 and 30, then they should seriously consider following the American Cancer Society's high risk for breast cancer recommendations: begin screening mammograms and Breast MRIs annually beginning at age 30 [23].

Genetic testing can be costly and have legal and ethical implications. Many people do not want others to know that they are at greater risk of breast cancer than others, especially employers. Many fear that they may not get the new job they applied for or keep their existing job, and/or be denied health insurance coverage. The Genetic Information Non-discrimination Act (GINA) of 2008 was passed for these very reasons. It protects people's privacy of genetic information and the diagnosis of a disease process from discrimination for patients in the United States. This law prevents insurance carriers from denying coverage and employers from requesting genetic information as part of the application requirement [24]. Patient confidentiality and consent for genetic testing remains a key concern for patients worried about access to their medical records. As such, part of GINA's role is to make a patient's genetic information fall under a special classification known as "health information" so that it would fall under the Health Insurance Portability and Accountability Act (HIPAA) of 2013 which frames the privacy requirements for genetic information and who has access [24].

For those that want to get evaluated for the BRCA1 & 2 gene, there are more reasonable options for testing compared to 10 years ago. Today, there are multiple private genetic testing companies that will send you a genetic test kit, that includes BRCA1 & 2 genetic testing, without a clinician's order for between $199 and up [25]. This allows women to self-refer if they do not want to go to genetic counseling before getting tested. With this ease of access to the public, clinicians need to be familiar with these tests, their interpretation, and devising an individualized plan of care based on the report findings since patients will turn to their healthcare provider for answers if the results are confusing [20].

Patient protections have been established through the creation of molecular tumor boards (MTB). These boards are designed to ensure patients receive appropriate cancer testing and treatments derived on the premise of evidence-based plans of care based on the type of cancer, and the most applicable and effective cancer treatments. The MTB assigns a physician-oncologist that is assigned to the patient's care and responsible for their testing, treatments, and outcomes. These treatments also include targeted gene therapy considerations based on the specific genetic mutation and molecular fusion [20, 26].

4. Common signs and symptoms for concern

There are many different signs and symptoms for breast cancer that range from a lump in the breast without pain to a lump in the breast with pain, peau d'orange skin, nipple discharge, dimpling or puckering of the breast tissue, and/or obvious changes in breast or nipple appearance (inversion), pain in the axillary region, asymmetry, or swollen lymph nodes of the upper arm leading into the tail of spence [27].

4.1 Lumps

Lumps in the breast that are nodular are more easily felt before a woman's menses and usually involves tenderness. Many women have breast fibroids that are easily palpable as well and are triggered by multiple factors: caffeine use, stress, intake of certain foods such as chocolate. When performing a clinical breast exam, be sure to document the location, size, shape, thickness, consistency (solid or fluid filled), whether the lump is fixed or moveable, tenderness, any recent changes and/or trauma to the breast as well. When assessing the tenderness of the breast, the type of pain should be determined. Is the pain focal, diffuse, or cyclic in nature [9].

4.2 Nipple discharge

Nipple discharge should be evaluated for its origin: physiologic or pathologic. Is the discharge a response to normal hormonal processes in the body such as pregnancy, stress, breast feeding, changes in sleeping habits, medication induced (birth control), and/or breast stimulation? If it is related to one of these situations then it is considered to be physiologic [1, 9]. Galactorrhea is milk production in the absence of pregnancy and may be caused by certain medications such as birth control, diuretics, corticosteroids, or digitalis [1]. If the nipple discharge is only on one side, has an abrupt presence of discharge, is related to a lump/mass on the side with a discharge, and/or is serous or bloody, then there is cause for concern. This type of nipple discharge is considered pathological in origin and warrants further workups to determine the cause [9].

4.3 Diagnostic screening

Diagnostic screening for lumps in the breast has a hierarchy of sorts that can be simplified in **Table 2**.

Diagnostic Screening	Age: 30 and over w/ BRCA1 or 2 mutation	Age: less than 40 w/ lump/ mass	Age: over 40 w/ lump/ mass	Age 40 and over w/ breast augmentation
Ultrasound		X		
Mammogram	X		X	X
Breast MRI	X			

Table 2.
Diagnostic scan recommendations by age and risk [23].

Women under 40 years of age with a lump/mass identified in their breast(s) requires a diagnostic ultrasound due to the denseness of the breast; however, women over 40 have less denseness and a diagnostic mammogram is warranted. When documenting where the lumps are found, use the face of a clock to identify the location of the lump and be sure to document the shape, size, consistency, and moveability of the lump of each corresponding lump when ordering the diagnostic mammogram or ultrasound. This information is helpful to the radiology facility [1].

Those with a known BRCA1 or 2 mutation should begin MRI and diagnostic mammogram screenings annually at age 30 to ensure early detection [23]. Maintaining a consistency with a specific radiology facility is important. Having one site where one's ultrasound, mammogram, and/or MRIs are completed provides a history of past scans which allows for comparison between the current ultrasound, MRI, or mammogram and past ultrasound, MRI, or mammograms to determine if there is a change in the breasts as well as the severity of the change from one year to the next (**Figure 4**) [20].

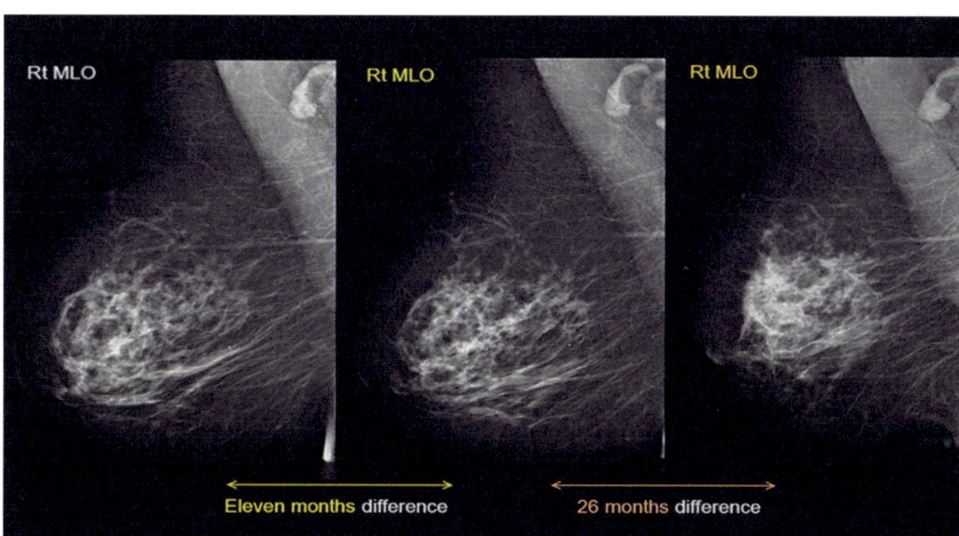

Figure 4.
Bilateral breast cancer radiologic pathologic correlation [28]. Permission granted to share this image compliments of Dr. László Tabár.

5. Breast cancer

Cancer is a mutation of healthy cells whose DNA was not repaired back to a homogenous status. This mutation is expressed through biomarkers and molecular subtypes that drive the severity and prognosis of said cancers [29]. The BRCA gene has gotten skewed in its role in breast cancer. Its primary role is to repair damaged DNA and is considered to be a tumor suppressor, but with a mutated form of this gene, it can cause breast cancer and this is what this gene is now known for, not its original function [30]. The BRCA1 & 2 gene mutation is one culprit of a familial genetic mutation identified through whole gene sequencing [31]. Patients can be evaluated for the BRCA1 & 2 mutation and know whether they carry this mutated form of the gene and take precautions to proactively screen more frequently and/or make informed decisions about their plan of care, options, and further testing for tumor markers. The individualized plan of care and having the knowledge that the risk is greater for breast cancer may assist in a more active role between the patient and their provider to ensure early detection remains the focus [29]. Why is this so important? Women with this mutation have a much higher risk of developing breast cancer compared to the general population without this genetic mutation (see **Table 3**). The Online Mendelain Inheritance in Man (OMIM) provides guidance on the BRCA1 & 2 gene phenotype relationship in relation to the chromosomal location, inheritance, mapping, and gene/locus (see **Table 4**). Also, women with a history of epithelial ovarian cancer should consider being tested for the BRCA gene mutation and any other cancer genes that align with ovarian cancer risk [30].

Over 80% of BRCA1 mutations lose its ability to differentiate breast stem cells and as a result it cannot express three specific receptors: human epidermal growth factor, estrogen, and progesterone. BRCA2 mutations have a higher rate of ovarian cancer compared to BRCA1 mutations. Studies have found that to reduce the risk of breast and/or ovarian cancer for those with either BRCA1 or 2 mutation is to proactively have an oophorectomy [33]. This could be due to the decline in hormone fluctuation, especially hormone receptor sensitive breast cancers.

5.1 Diagnostic testing, prognosis, and susceptibility

There are advanced diagnostic testing options rooted in next-generation sequencing technology that is available when testing for specific breast cancer mutations. Clinicians can order these tests once a diagnosis of breast cancer is determined. These include the following: next-generation sequencing (NGS), sequenced analytic data pipelines derived from NGS, anchored multiplex polymerase chain reaction (AMP) also derived from NGS. Other tests that determine the aggressive nature of the cancer, its recurrence risk, and what adjuvant therapies are needed based on genetic analysis:

Breast cancer	Percentage who gets breast cancer over a lifetime up to between age 70–80
BRCA1 mutation positive	55–72%
BRCA2 mutation positive	45–69%
General population without BRCA gene mutation	13%

Table 3.
Percentage of breast cancer patient comparisons [30].

Gene / locus	Gene/locus MIM #	Phenotype: familial, breast-ovarian cancer	Phenotype map	Phenotype MIM #	Inheritance: autosomal dominant	Inheritance: multifactorial	Chromosomal location
BRCA1	113,705	Yes	3	604,370	Yes	Yes	17q21.31
BRCA2	600,185	Yes	3	612,555	Yes	No	13q13.1
RAD51C	602,774	Yes, susceptibility to, 3	3	613,399			17q22
RAD51D	602,954	Yes, susceptibility to, 4	3	614,291			17q12
TP53		Breast cancer	1				17p13.3

MIM = Mendelian Inheritance in Man. Phenotype map legend: 1 = underlying defect unknown, but mapped; 2 = mapped with statistical methods; 3 = disorder's molecular basis is known; and 4 = multiple gene involvement.

Table 4.
Breast cancer phenotype-gene correlation [32–36].

Test detections	BRCA1 & 2	Next-generation sequencing	Sequenced analytic data pipelines	Anchored multiplex polymerase chain reaction
BRCA gene mutation	X	X	X	X
DNA variant		X	X	X
DNA fusion		X	X	X
Adjuvant therapy susceptibility		X	X	X

Table 5.
Breast cancer testing considerations [20, 37].

(1) MammaPrint uses 70 genes to test for prognosis and the adjuvant therapy susceptibility and (2) Oncotype DX Breast Recurrence Score Test uses a 21 gene scoring system to determine cancer recurrence, cancer aggression, and susceptibility to adjuvant therapy [20]. All of these tests provide a different function/use in testing that varies from identifying if cancer is present at all to specific breast cancer variants, instability, fusion of DNA, and/or identifying specific markers that make the cancer cells more susceptible and responsive to adjuvant treatment modalities [20]. The most advanced tests identify the rearrangement of chromosomal intergenic fusion (see **Table 5**). Both types of genetic mutations, germline and somatic can be individually fused or a mix of both and can be found in later stages of metastatic cancers [20]. Specific fusions are associated with molecular subtype ER+ metastatic cancers in the later cancer stages [20]. One promising test that can be done with NGS is to profile the cancer and its susceptibility of adjuvant therapy for cell-free DNA (cfDNA) found in plasma [37]. Circulating tumor DNA (ctDNA) are also found in plasma and helps to determine the risk of recurrence of cancer after remission [38].

The type of biomarkers and molecular subtypes play a significant role in the tumor growth and prognosis of this type of breast cancer (see **Table 6**).

Early detection/diagnosis of breast cancer is crucial in determining treatment plans and improving the chance for a positive response to treatments to achieve remission. Those that are diagnosed with a localized early-stage breast cancer (in situ) is 66% [10]. The five-year survival rate for the different stages when diagnosed is as follows: localized breast cancer = 99%, regional breast cancer = 86%, and distant breast cancer = 30% [10]. Invasive breast cancer is cancer that has spread through the blood or lymph nodes to other parts of the body, also known as metastasis. The percentage of breast cancers that are invasive is 83% [10]. This number is alarming and the advancements in targeted gene and immunotherapy are new tools in fighting breast cancer and improving survival rates [10, 20].

5.2 Treatment options

Traditional cancer treatments are chemotherapy, radiation therapy, hormone blocking therapy, and surgery (lumpectomy or mastectomy). Patients with a mastectomy may consider breast reconstruction surgery and should discuss this with their surgeon about when would be the best time to undergo this type of procedure based on their treatment plan [10]. Chemotherapy and hormone therapy has been around for a long time; however, the next promising therapies to impact treatment

	Estrogen Receptor (ER) + (HR+)		**Hormone Receptor Negative (HR−)**	**HR-**
Molecular subtype	**HER2- (Luminal A)**	**HER2+ (Luminal B) Ki61**	**HER2+ (ER−, HER2−, PR−) triple negative breast cancer (TNBC) basal-subtype**	**HER2+ (enriched)**
% of all breast cancers	68%	10%	10%	4%
Growth of tumor	Slow	Fast	Aggressive	Aggressive
Prognosis	Good	Poor	Poor	Improved w/ targeted gene therapy
Cancer cell grade	Lower	Higher	Higher	Higher
5-year survival rate	94%	91%	85%	77%

Table 6.
Breast cancer biomarkers and molecular subtypes [10].

modalities include non-viral targeted gene therapy and immunotherapy. These cutting edge therapies joined the fight against breast cancer as adjuvant therapy, usually in combination with traditional therapies [10]. In pursuit of treating patients with the most effective treatment allowed, one such newcomer over the last few years has been precision therapy where oncogene drivers are used in individualized treatments using the molecular makeup of the patient to combat cancer cells with targeted gene therapy [20]. The impact of molecular subtypes on treatment and patient outcomes is reflected in **Table 7**. Immunotherapy is an innovative approach in fighting breast cancer by using one's own immune system to target and kill cancer cells. This type of therapy is called checkpoint inhibitors and is being used for TNBC.

The molecular subtype represents the hormone receptor status for estrogen, progesterone, and human epidermal growth receptor 2 (HER2). Based on the hormone receptor affinity, you can see the correlation for subtype, the Ki-67 recurrence predictor for cell division/replication, prognosis, therapy type, and treatment options. TNBC has the poorest prognosis, but recent clinical trials have proved positive in slowing the progression of metastatic or recurring TNBC, although some side effects are worse than traditional therapies. Sacituzumab Govitecan (Trodelvy) is a drug approved by the FDA in 2021 and is showing great promise for TNBC patients [41].

There are other new innovative research studies that have found that breast cancer stem cells (CSC) can achieve apoptosis with the use of specific PDE4 inhibitors (anti-inflammatory medications) [42]. One study found that there is a signaling pathway to turn on cancer stem cells to survive through upregulation of PI3K/AKT/mTOR which increase CSC levels and in turn increases PDE4 levels. If these pathways can be turned on then they can be turned off. In turning off the pathway, it can stop the cyclic adenosine monophosphate (cAMP) from binding to regulatory subunits of inactive protein kinase A (PKA); thereby, stopping the conversion to an active form of (PKA) to trigger AKT and mTOR. Turning off this pathway will turn on autophagy of CSC and lead to cell death of the cancer cell. This cascade of signaling pathways is crucial

Molecular subtype	HER2– Luminal A	HER2+/ PR+/– Luminal B	TNBC	HER2+Enriched
HR+/–	Estrogen+/ PR+	Estrogen+/ PR+	HR–/PR–/HER2–	HR–/PR–
Ki-67 proliferative index/recurrence predictor	</equal 14%	>/equal 14%	Any	Any
Prognosis	Good/slow	Poor/fast	Poor/highly aggressive w/ metastasis	Poor/highly aggressive
Therapy type	Estrogen deprivation	Estrogen deprivation	Precision therapy	Precision therapy
Oncogenic fusion therapy resistance	Increased risk	Increased risk	Need further susceptible pathways for effective treatment	Need further susceptible pathways for effective treatment
Treatment plan to fusion/ mutation	Combination therapy	Combination therapy	Combination therapy	Combination therapy

Table 7.
Molecular subtypes on treatment and outcomes [20, 39, 40].

in stopping phosphatidylinositol-3-kinase (PI3K) from proliferating CSC growth. CSCs were found to have elevated PDE4 levels when compared to healthy stem cells. Thus, the use of PDE4 inhibitors may hold the key to the downregulation of PI3K/ AKT pathway, thus reducing resistance to chemotherapy in CSCs [42]. This study found that PKA and cAMP levels antagonized the signaling pathway "PI3K/AKT/ mTOR" and caused "cell cycle arrest" [42].

5.3 Breast cancer incidence, mortality rate, and the disparity gap

The disparity gap for breast cancer incidence is not what one might expect with Caucasians having the highest breast cancer incidence rate followed by Black women per every 100,000 women in the United States (see **Table 8**). The mortality rate is similarly surprising with Asian women having the lowest mortality rate and Hispanic women having the second lowest mortality rate compared to Caucasian women with the third lowest mortality rate, whereas Black women had the highest mortality rate. Accordingly, between 2012 and 2018, there was a 9% disparity gap between Black women compared to Caucasian and Asian Pacific Island women for a 5-year relative survival rate, 83% vs. 92%. This difference in survival rate translates into more

Breast cancer rate per 100,000	Caucasian	Black	Native American	Asian	Hispanic
Incidence	133.7	127.8	111.3	101.3	99.2
Mortality	19.7	27.6	20.5	11.7	13.7

Table 8.
Breast cancer incidence and mortality rates by ethnicity in the US from 2016 to 2020 [10].

deaths in black women across the spectrum due to differences in access to care and insurance coverage/financial ability to pay for treatments [10]. The disparity gap for breast cancer survivors with late-stage breast cancer (stage 4) has begun to decrease steadily. This disparity gap has been zeroed out among racial/ethnic groups as a result of the Medicaid expansion programs implemented over the last couple of years [10]. Survival rates that are consistent with the elimination of disparity gaps will continue to take time, but as noted in late-stage breast cancers, this too is achievable.

Five percent of breast cancer survivors will face the daunting diagnosis of cancer once more after remission. When looking at the recurrence of breast cancer in women, there is a 70% chance that it will be in the opposite breast (contralateral). One study's findings reported that black women had a 44% greater chance of this recurrence whereas Hispanic women had an 11% greater chance of the same recurrence in the opposite breast compared to their Caucasian counterparts [10].

6. Conclusion

The breast, in many ways, defines a young girl's journey into womanhood, motherhood, and old age, ever changing along the way [1]. With older age being one of the main risk factors for breast cancer and the changes that come with aging, it provides insight into the body's own shortcomings physically and genetically. Breast cancer impacts patients in many ways: physically, financially, emotionally, and functionally; however, advanced technologies in genomics through mapping of the human genome, next-generation sequencing, and evidence-based treatments all combined is helping to unlock the mystery of many disease processes, including breast cancer. This innovative science is changing the course of how we see, treat, and think about patient care, outcomes, and what is possible. The more we learn, the more impact we can have on patient care, treatment plans, and improved patient outcomes. We are on the cusp of a new scientific era, but new advancements in breast cancer treatments are still needed to continually strive to cure cancer for today's cancer patients and future generations to come [20].

Conflict of interest

The authors declare no conflict of interest.

Author details

Tammy Walker-Smith
Texas A&M University Corpus Christi, Corpus Christi, TX, United States of America

*Address all correspondence to: tammy.walker-smith@tamucc.edu

IntechOpen

© 2023 The Author(s). Licensee IntechOpen. This chapter is distributed under the terms of the Creative Commons Attribution License (http://creativecommons.org/licenses/by/3.0), which permits unrestricted use, distribution, and reproduction in any medium, provided the original work is properly cited. (cc) BY

References

[1] Jarvis C. Physical Examination and Health Assessment. 7th ed. St. Louis, Missouri: W. B. Saunders; 2016

[2] Dains, J.E., L.C. Baumann, and P. Scheibel, Advanced Health Assessment and Clinical Diagnosis in Primary Care. 6th ed. 2020, St. Louis, Missouri, Elsevier

[3] Lynch PM. Breast Anatomy Normal Scheme, B.A.N. Scheme, Editor. 2006. Cc BY 3.0

[4] Memorial Sloan Kettering Cancer Center. Anatomy of the Breast. 2023. Available from: https://www.mskcc.org/cancer-care/types/breast/anatomy-breast

[5] Pillay J, Davis TJ. Physiology, lactation. In: StatPearls. StatPearls Publishing LLC: Treasure Island (FL); 2023

[6] Cancer Research UK; Wikipedia Commons, Lymph Nodes in and Around the Breast, L.N.i.a.A.t. Breast, Editor. 2016

[7] Society, AC Lymph Nodes and Cancer. 2023. Available from: https://www.cancer.org/cancer/diagnosis-staging/lymph-nodes-and-cancer.html

[8] Sattari M, Serwint JR, Levine DM. Maternal implications of breastfeeding: A review for the internist. The American Journal of Medicine. 2019;**132**(8):912-920

[9] Bickley L. Bates' Guide to Physical Examination and History Taking. 13th ed. Philadelphia, PA: Wolters Kluwer; 2021

[10] American Cancer Society. Breast Cancer Facts and Figures: 2022-2024. GA: Atlanta; 2022

[11] Li CM et al. Aging-associated alterations in mammary epithelia and stroma revealed by single-cell RNA sequencing. Cell Reports. 2020;**33**(13):108566

[12] Mantovani A. The inflammation—Cancer connection. The FEBS Journal. 2018;**285**(4):638-640

[13] Huelse JM et al. MERTK in cancer therapy: Targeting the receptor tyrosine kinase in tumor cells and the immune system. Pharmacology & Therapeutics. 2020;**213**:107577

[14] U.S. Preventive Services Task Force. Final Update Summary: BRCA Related Cancer: Risk Assessment, Genetic Counseling, and Genetic Testing. 2016. Available from: https://www.uspreventiveservicestaskforce.org/Page/Document/UpdateSummaryFinal/brca-related-cancer-risk-assessment-genetic-counseling-and-genetic-testing

[15] National Breast Cancer Foundation. Breast Self-Exam. 2023. Available from: https://www.nationalbreastcancer.org/breast-self-exam/

[16] U. S. Preventive Services Task Force. Breast cancer screening. 2016. Available from: https://www.uspreventiveservicestaskforce.org/Page/Document/UpdateSummaryFinal/breast-cancer-screening

[17] Banegas MP et al. Evaluating breast cancer risk projections for Hispanic women. Breast Cancer Research and Treatment. 2012;**132**(1):1-11

[18] Walker-Smith TL, Baldwin S. A quality improvement initiative: Improving mammogram screening rates among low-income Hispanic women

in primary care. Journal of Doctoral Nursing Practice. 2020;**13**(1):71-78

[19] National Cancer Institute. Breast Cancer Risk Assessment Tool: Risk Calculator. 2023. Available from: https://bcrisktool.cancer.gov/calculator.html

[20] Walker-Smith TL, Peck J. Genetic and genomic advances in breast cancer diagnosis and treatment. Nursing for Women's Health. 2019;**23**(6):518-525

[21] Haas JS et al. Provider attitudes and screening practices following changes in breast and cervical cancer screening guidelines. Journal of General Internal Medicine. 2016;**31**(1):52-59

[22] Gabram SGA et al. Assessing breast cancer risk and providing treatment recommendations: Immediate impact of an educational session. Breast Journal. 2009;**15**:39-45

[23] Susan G. Komen. Breast Cancer Screening for Women at Higher Risk. 2022. Available from: https://www.komen.org/breast-cancer/screening/when-to-screen/high-risk-women/

[24] National Human Genome Research Institute. Genetic Discrimination. 2022. Available from: https://www.genome.gov/about-genomics/policy-issues/Genetic-Discrimination

[25] 23andme. Health+Ancestry Service. 2023. Available from: https://www.23andme.com/dna-health-ancestry/

[26] Merry D et al. Trust and responsibility in molecular tumour boards. Bioethics. 2018;**32**(7):464-472

[27] American Cancer Society. Breast Cancer Signs and symptoms. 2023. Available from: https://www.cancer.org/cancer/types/breast-cancer/screening-tests-and-early-detection/breast-cancer-signs-and-symptoms.html

[28] Global Radiology CME. Bilateral Breast Cancer Radiologic Pathologic Correlation. 2017. Available from: https://static.wixstatic.com/media/e35976_5474bc88964c430cb8cdb27282344b1d~mv2.png/v1/fill/w_1000,h_743,al_c,usm_0.66_1.00_0.01/e35976_5474bc88964c430cb8cdb27282344b1d~mv2.png

[29] Walker-Smith T, Murphey C, Peck JL, CME. Addressing whole-genome sequencing and breast cancer in primary care. Clinical Advisor. 2019;**22**(1):24-31

[30] Institute, N.C. BRCA Gene Mutations: Cancer Risk and Genetic Testing. 2020. Available from: https://www.cancer.gov/about-cancer/causes-prevention/genetics/brca-fact-sheet

[31] Sokolenko AP et al. Identification of novel hereditary cancer genes by whole exome sequencing. Cancer Letters. 2015;**369**(2):274-288

[32] Online Mendelian Inheritance in Man Breast-ovarian Cancer, Familial, Susceptibility to, 1; BROVCA1. 2016. Available from: http://omim.org/entry/604370?search=BRCA1&highlight=brca1

[33] Online Mendelian Inheritance in Man. Breast-ovarian Cancer, Familial, Susceptibility to, 2; BROVCA2. 2016. Available from: http://omim.org/entry/612555?search=BRCA2&highlight=brca2

[34] OMIM. Breast-Ovarian Cancer, Familial, Susceptibility to, 3; BROVCA3. 2021. Available from: https://www.omim.org/entry/613399?search=Breast%20cancer&highlight=breast%20cancer%20cancerous

[35] OMIM. Breast-Ovarian Cancer, Familial, Susceptibility to, 4; BROVCA4.

2011. Available from: https://www.omim.org/entry/614291

[36] OMIM. Breast Cancer-Related Regulator of TP53. 2017. Available from: https://www.omim.org/entry/113721?search=Breast%20cancer&highlight=breast%20cancer%20cancerous

[37] Esposito, Abate R et al. Next generation sequencing-based profiling of cell free DNA in patients with advanced non-small cell lung cancer: Advantages and pitfalls. Cancers (Basel). 2020;**12**(12):2-3

[38] Niravath P, Cakar B, Ellis M. The role of genetic testing in the selection of therapy for breast cancer. JAMA Oncology. 2017;**3**(2):262-268

[39] Chiu AM et al. Integrative analysis of the inter-tumoral heterogeneity of triple-negative breast cancer. Scientific Reports. 2018;**8**:11807

[40] Mohammed AA. The clinical behavior of different molecular subtypes of breast cancer. Cancer Treatment and Research Communications. 2021;**29**:100469

[41] Loibl S et al. Health-related quality of life in the phase III ASCENT trial of sacituzumab govitecan versus standard chemotherapy in metastatic triple-negative breast cancer. European Journal of Cancer. 2023;**178**:23-33

[42] Mukherjee P et al. PDE4 inhibitor eliminates breast cancer stem cells via noncanonical activation of mTOR. Journal of Cellular Biochemistry. 2022;**123**(12):1980-1996

Chapter 2

Screening, Surveillance, and Survivorship after Breast Reconstruction

Karinn Chambers

Abstract

In this chapter the recommendations for breast cancer screening, surveillance, and survivorship after breast reconstructive surgery will be discussed. The average risk patient, high risk patient, and the breast cancer survivor after breast reconstruction of any form will be outlined with pertinent challenges, complications, and patient related concerns detailed. The lifestyle changes and psychosocial concerns of patients after breast reconstructive surgery will also be described. The patient's journey is the central theme of this chapter, as are the surgical choices they make and how that might affect their future care.

Keywords: screening, surveillance, survivorship, risk assessment, breast cancer

1. Introduction

When a patient with a breast related concern is faced with challenging discussions regarding breast reconstruction options, there are many variables that must factor into the decision making process. Risk assessment should be performed so that the patient can understand if they are at average risk for breast cancer or at an elevated risk based on quantitative risk assessment models. The indications for surgery should also be fully understood as that can affect the options available to the patient. Any treatments that may be required after surgery should also factor into the decision making process. Once breast reconstruction has been performed it has the potential to alter screening, surveillance, and survivorship recommendations and the patient, the surgical oncologist, and the plastic surgeon must be prepared for those challenges.

In order to facilitate the decision making process all the ramifications of breast reconstruction must be disclosed to the patient and the patient care team. In this chapter the recommendations for breast cancer screening, surveillance, and survivorship will be discussed. The average risk patient, high risk patient, and the breast cancer survivor after breast reconstruction of any form will be outlined with pertinent challenges, complications, and patient related concerns detailed. The lifestyle changes and psychosocial concerns of patients after breast reconstructive surgery will also be described. The patient's journey is the central theme of this chapter, as are the surgical choices they make and how that will affect their future care.

2. The average risk patient

One in eight women will develop breast cancer. This correlates with an approximately 12% average risk that a woman will develop breast cancer in their lifetime. A woman may decide to proceed with breast reconstruction in varying forms and for many different reasons. In the non-cancer setting breast reconstruction can take the form of breast augmentation, fat grafting, tissue transfers, or silicone injections. These interventions may seem indolent to the patient, but to the surgical oncologist and the breast radiologist even these benign procedures can lead to challenges in future breast cancer screening.

If a patient chooses to undergo a breast procedure of any kind they must be informed that this will lead to changes in the architecture of the breast. Injection of any material into the breast can lead to internal changes and scarring that can be hard to differentiate from a malignant lesion. This finding may then need to be biopsied to determine its true pathological derivation. The anxiety that surrounds a callback for abnormal imaging and the need for a breast biopsy is substantial and should be taken into account. Injection of a foreign material into the breast can lead to pronounced inflammatory changes, including a cellulitis of the breast necessitating treatment with antibiotics and steroids. The treatment of these findings and subsequent breast changes also have consequences to be considered.

A patient who undergoes breast augmentation will still need to undergo screening mammography in order to provide early cancer detection. For the patient with breast implants who needs to undergo routine screening mammography there are some special concerns that should be noted. Patients who have implants are often concerned that the mammogram itself will rupture them, and this is not true. What does need to be considered is that it becomes increasingly more challenging to compress the breast appropriately for the patient with breast implants and all the breast tissue may not be seen clearly. The tissue near the implant will be hard to compress and thus achieve the magnification necessary to see the calcifications or architectural distortion that may indicate an abnormality. Approximately 20% of a patient's breast tissue may not be visualized well after breast augmentation when undergoing screening for breast cancer.

Patients who have a family history of breast cancer who do not meet the criteria of a high risk patient may choose to have a prophylactic mastectomy with reconstruction. That reconstruction could be either implant based or with autologous tissue transfers. Which form of reconstruction is appropriate must be decided on a case by case basis in regards to that patient's particular history and concerns with the surgical oncologist ensuring that the patient understands all the risks associated with these prophylactic procedures. The recommendations for further care in this setting will be discussed in the section related to high risk patients as they would be similar.

The recommendations for screening of the patient at average risk for breast cancer include yearly mammography after the age of 40. This is recommended to continue until the age of 75 or at which time 10 yrs. or less of life expectancy is estimated [1]. The aforementioned breast changes with difficulty in the establishment of a benign or malignant lesion and subsequent need for a tissue diagnosis can lead to mental and physical discomfort in the fear and anxiety that this can provoke, as well as in the procedure itself. Patients should be counseled accordingly prior to breast reconstruction as to the risks involved, and that this may lead to additional breast findings and breast biopsies in the future.

3. The high risk patient

A patient who's risk for breast cancer has been assessed and whose risk is greater than or equal to 20% is classified as a patient at high risk for breast cancer. These assessments are made based on models such as the Gail Model or Tyrer-Cusick Model of risk assessment. In these models the patient's hormonal history, breast history, and family history of breast and/or ovarian cancer are utilized to estimate that individual's lifetime risk for breast cancer. It can thus be understood that with an elevated risk for breast cancer and with family members who have undergone treatment for breast cancer that the patient may want to do everything they can to prevent this from occurring. High risk screening paradigms as well as prophylactic procedures are then discussed with these patients, as well as genetic testing for predispositions to cancer where appropriate [2].

If an individual who is at elevated risk for breast cancer does not wish to undergo prophylactic/preventive surgery, most often in the form of a bilateral mastectomy, they will be followed closely according to the guidelines documented for that patient population. High risk screening includes two clinical exams yearly as well as annual mammography and annual MRI [2]. Many providers and surgical oncologists will recommend that the patient stagger the recommended breast imaging at six month intervals so that they do not proceed with a year between these imaging modalities and can be seen twice a year with new imaging available at that visit.

When the decision has been made to proceed with prophylactic bilateral mastectomy the patient must first understand that this does not mean that they could never get breast cancer. Surgical intervention has been documented to decrease the risk of breast cancer development by 90%, but that risk is not zero. The patient is then given the option of undergoing immediate breast reconstruction or delayed breast reconstruction. If the patient desires breast reconstruction they then must choose which type of reconstruction they would like to have. Typically the choice is between an implant based reconstruction or autologous tissue transfer.

With an implant based reconstruction the common challenges noted post-operatively include implant rupture (approximately 4% risk in the first 2 years post-operatively and nearly 50% at 10 yrs), capsular contracture, rippling of the skin, and migration/flipping of the implant. In many settings a temporary tissue expander implant is used to stretch the skin post operatively so that an appropriate breast size can be reached, necessitating additional surgery for the final stage of reconstruction. Breast implants are not meant to last the entire life-span of the patient and often need to be replaced after 10 yrs. in vivo. Another more recent concern has been documented in cases of implant associated B-Cell lymphoma, mainly in regard to textured implants placed 8–10 yrs. ago [3].

For the patients who undergo autologous tissue transfers as part of their breast reconstruction, the following should be discussed. It should be noted that the site where the donor tissue is to be removed from is separate and at risk for its own set of complications. The overall failure rate of these reconstructive techniques can be quoted at 1–3% with a wound infection rate estimated at 5–12% [4]. The gravity of these surgeries should be relayed, and the prolonged recovery time explored. These surgeries are often discussed as a one-step surgery, in that there is no required second step to complete the reconstruction, but many patients undergo additional minor procedures to obtain the cosmetic result desired.

After autologous tissue transfer breast reconstruction, it should also be stated that the scarring and internal remodeling of that tissue can take a quite prolonged course and that the patient might note changes to the consistency of that tissue months after surgery. This is most commonly seen in areas of fat necrosis that develop in the autologous tissue, presenting like abnormal chest wall masses that can be quite concerning for a breast malignancy, requiring further diagnostic evaluation and potentially biopsies of that area. In the patient who is at elevated risk for breast cancer the additional changes after autologous tissue transfer reconstruction that may be noted and need further evaluation should be explored in pre-operative discussions to prevent undo anxiety and ensure that they get proper care should a new finding be discovered.

4. The breast cancer survivor

In the case of the breast cancer survivor the first step in delivery of their care may be recognizing that these patients are facing a traumatic experience and that their ability to make decision may be hampered by anxiety, denial, shock, along with difficulty understanding the complexity of breast cancer care. Additional time to make these life altering decisions can be useful in this instance to allow for time to process the diagnosis and treatment options, to talk to other family members and loved ones who can assist them through this process, and to seek second opinions if desired to ensure the patient understands what they are facing. Additional office visits may be necessary to review the options or talk to additional care givers if the patient is noted to be struggling with the decision on how best to proceed. A patient must be able to develop a sense of trust in their surgical team prior to proceeding and the time necessary to establish this is quite variable.

When the surgical plan for the breast cancer patient is devised, and all the options have been explored, if the patient proceeds with unilateral or bilateral mastectomy with reconstruction there are pre-operative, peri-operative, and post-operative considerations to be disclosed. Pre-operative concerns to be addressed include the timing of surgery, pre-operative risk stratification, as well as a clear delineation of all the risks and benefits to this approach. It should be noted here that according to current guidelines the surgical oncologist is recommended not to encourage prophylactic contralateral mastectomy for the breast cancer patient in the setting of no genetic predisposition to cancer as this greatly increases the surgical risks involved with very little risk reduction, as the risk of contralateral breast cancer is quoted at 0.4% per year [5].

4.1 The pre-operative breast Cancer patient

Current standard of care dictates that we should pursue surgical intervention within 30 days of the diagnosis of cancer. With the addition of the consultation with the plastic surgeon and the coordination of multiple surgical calendars, this can be quite challenging to obtain. Working together to obtain the earliest surgical date possible becomes incredibly important. Risk stratification in regards to cardiac clearance, pulmonary optimization, and renal status should also be factored into the process for those patients who require it. Any additional imaging, staging studies, genetic testing, and any other pre-operative referrals should be expedited as much as possible. The need for pre-operative systemic therapy must also be taken into consideration when treating a breast cancer patient. In the modern era pre-operative chemotherapy and immunotherapy are commonly used to treat triple negative breast cancer and Her-2 neu targeted therapies are used to treat Her-2 neu (+) breast cancer when appropriate. Neo-adjuvant chemotherapy prior to surgery in this setting is associated with a 60% compete pathological response rate, and the pathological response rate noted is then used to dictate further systemic treatment. The breast care team, with the keystone being the breast cancer care navigator, are integral to ensuring that the pre-operative process is facilitated as much as possible. Working with the patient through each step of the journey so that they are aware of how the process is unfolding is critical during this very stressful point in their life. Clear expectations of what to expect will help the patient immensely as they navigate their care.

4.2 The peri-operative breast cancer patient

Peri-operatively the expected hospital course, pain management, wound care, drain care, recovery experience, and post-operative limitations should be clearly delineated. If able the psychological aspects of losing a breast, or both breasts, should be approached with the patient as well. Many institutions have a policy in place where a patient is discharged to home on the day of their procedure if they are undergoing implant based reconstruction. In this setting it can be incredibly helpful to have a staff member call the patient the day after the procedure to ensure no complications have been noted post-operatively. Clear instructions on what to expect as well as what to look out for are usually provided by the physician or surgical facility of choice to assist with this. If the patient undergoes a period of 23 hour post-operative observation many of these concerns can be evaluated and readdressed prior to their discharge the following morning. After autologous tissue reconstruction patients are often admitted to the hospital with lengths of stay approximating three to five days.

Pain management is another critical component of the peri-operative discussion. Many great strides in multi-modal pain management have been documented and should be applied where appropriate. Multi-modal pain management can include Tylenol, NSAIDS, and muscle relaxants; in addition to local nerve blocks to lesson or alleviate the need for post-operative narcotics. Many patients voice anxiety concerning the level of pain that they are going to experience after surgery and they can be comforted that a pain management approach that attempts to control pain from many different angles will be used.

Drain care, post-operative wound care, and any specific limitations should also be addressed in the peri-operative phase. What the recovery period after unilateral or bilateral mastectomy may look like is another essential component of these discussions. A recovery period of approximately 30 days is not unreasonable. Drains that remain in place for 2–3 weeks is not uncommon. Bathing restrictions while the drains are present is often noted as well as lifting restrictions for up to four to six weeks post-operatively. There are often physicians who prescribe antibiotics post-operatively for the time frame in which the drains remain in place as well. Working with the nursing staff who provides this information to the patient to ensure that it is correct and that the patient is able to assimilate this information is essential to decreasing the incidence of post-operative complications noted, such as; hematoma/seroma formation, infection, and other wound related complications, while ensuring their compliance with the instructions.

After discussions in the pre and peri-operative phase of the breast cancer patient's surgical care it may be noted that they might benefit from additional assistance. A psychologist or social worker may need to be involved if the patient requires additional resources to cope with the psychosocial aspects of their health.

A physical therapist may be required to assist with return to full range of motion as the patient recovers. For the elderly or infirm a subacute nursing facility may be necessary to assist with their daily activities until they improve and are able to return to their baseline health status. A holistic approach to the individual patient and their care is necessary to achieve the best outcome and can require a multidisciplinary approach.

4.3 The post-operative breast cancer patient

The breast cancer patient's journey into survivorship often is felt to begin in the post-operative period. For the patient who chooses to undergo mastectomy with reconstruction that journey begins with accepting an entirely new body image; and for a woman, the loss of an organ very deeply tied into their gender identity, sexuality, and maternal nature. From a technical perspective long term complications after mastectomy and reconstruction include numbness to the skin of the mastectomy flaps, loss of the nipple areolar complex in many cases, post-operative pain, and lymphedema. If adjuvant radiation is required after mastectomy with reconstruction this can increase the risk of lymphedema noted as well as the previously described risks of capsular contracture and skin rippling after implant reconstruction. In general the skin sparred at time of mastectomy can become darker, thicker, and have decreased wound healing capabilities. All these aspects can be combined into a cosmetic result that is less pleasing then imagined prior. The risk of a patient's breast cancer diagnosis necessitating adjuvant radiation should thus be broached to allow for complete disclosure, often leading to a recommendation for delayed reconstruction should that risk be high.

In the post-operative period there also remains a risk that the patient will develop a wound infection or wound dehiscence, leading to implant removal for those patients who chose to undergo an implant based reconstruction. For the patient who undergoes a nipple sparing mastectomy there is a noted risk of loss of the nipple areolar complex. The mastectomy flaps themselves are at risk of ischemia and thus tissue loss that may require debridement, skin grafting, or other procedures not excluding removal of the implant to allow for wound closure and another attempt at delayed reconstruction. In the patient who undergoes autologous tissue transfer reconstruction, as noted prior, the wound related challenges discussed also apply to the site of tissue harvest. If abdominal muscle is taken at time of autologous tissue transfer this infers an associated risk of abdominal wall hernia formation that should be taken into consideration.

In the peri-operative to immediately post-operative period after autologous tissue reconstruction there is a risk that the whole tissue graft will be lost should a post-operative complication occur, such as venous outflow obstruction or arterial occlusion. In certain settings leeches can be and have been applied to the reconstructed breast flap in an attempt to alleviate venous congestion and preserve graft function. This would be quite a troubling and unexpected event to the patient who is unaware that this is a potential outcome. In the setting of autologous tissue transfer reconstruction it can be also noted that areas of fat necrosis can develop that can be quite large and concerning. Tissue contracture may occur to a degree that necessitates fat grafting or other surgical approaches to filling the defect that remains. Multiple procedures may be necessary to achieve the final outcome desired and close clinical follow up is often required during this period to ensure optimal outcomes and that a recurrent cancer does not develop.

5. Life after breast reconstruction

The long-term effects of breast reconstruction after mastectomy in the prophylactic setting or in the breast cancer patient must also be mentioned at this time, as they are quite significant. The long-term outcomes these patients must contend with include physical and psychosocial concerns. The physical ramifications of breast reconstruction include but are not limited to; post mastectomy pain, long-term surveillance of the reconstructed breast, continued maintenance of the reconstructed breast, and decisions around nipple reconstruction/tattooing. The psychosocial aspects include loss of self, loss of sexual identity, loss of libido, and inability to connect with their partner physically and emotionally.

In regard to the physical components of life after breast reconstruction, post mastectomy pain may be the most common complaint noted among patients. Physical therapy, injections with local anesthetics, muscle relaxants, and medications for nerve pain can be used to assist in control of these symptoms. If the nipple areolar complex was removed at time of surgery, a decision must be made as to whether or not the patient would like to proceed with reconstruction of the nipple areolar complex. This may be performed via multiple different techniques, including 3-D tattooing. The long-term maintenance of the reconstructed breast previously mentioned can include things such as fat grafting and tissue transfers should areas of deficit be noted. Should the patient undergo an implant base reconstruction and reach the shelf life of that implant, the implants may need to be replaced. Long term maintenance of the reconstructed breast can also include further evaluation if new concerns develop, imaging of new findings with appropriate tissue diagnosis if necessary, and biopsy of areas of fat necrosis contained within the breast reconstructed with autologous tissue. Revision of the reconstruction may be required based on the cosmetic changes that appear overtime.

Long-term surveillance of the reconstructed breast and evaluation for cancer recurrence entails clinical exams at the discretion of the medical oncologist and surgical oncologist. This frequently means clinical exams every three to four months for the first two years and biannual exams between the second and fifth year after diagnosis. Yearly breast exams at the very least to follow. There would be no need for screening mammography to be performed after bilateral mastectomy with reconstruction, though imaging may be used in the diagnostic setting to work up a new breast related complaint.

The psychosocial ramifications for the patient after mastectomy with breast reconstruction are much harder to elicit and to quantify. Many if not most patients do not feel comfortable discussing with their doctors the most intimate aspects of their personal lives. It is noted however that many woman who have undergone these procedures have trouble with a negative body image, feeling that they are hideous to themselves and others post-operatively. They can sometimes feel less than human in losing a part of themselves. They can certainly feel like they have lost an essential part of what makes them a woman, harming their sense of gender and sexual identity. Physical intimacy with a significant other or spouse is a challenge for these individuals and many of them do not engage with their loved ones on that level for a prolonged period of time. A woman's breasts are also deeply rooted in their maternal nature as well and that loss can be devastating to a young woman looking to having children or with young children at home [6, 7].

Patients who are facing the decision to undergo or who have had a mastectomy with reconstruction are then faced with feelings of anxiety, confusion, fear, and often depression. The loss of a breast can leave a woman feeling that they will never be seen as beautiful again. If they are unmarried they might feel that they will never find a husband, get married, and have children as they had hoped. Those with spouses or significant others may feel that they will be viewed as unattractive and untouchable and continue the spiral into a lack of desire for intimacy. In addition, for the many woman whom anti-estrogen therapies are recommended, they may suffer from side effects that further decrease their libido and may actually make intimacy painful. Pre-operative, post-operative, and survivorship resources should be offered in counseling, psychological therapy, support groups, and management of treatment related side effects to ease the journey [6, 7].

6. Conclusion

The journey for the patient with a breast related concern or breast cancer that includes breast reconstruction is one that is delicate to navigate. The path forward must be directed by that individual as it is a very personal one. Though they may have many care givers, family members, and/or friends who are full of opinions, only the individual involved can even begin to fathom how the outcome will affect them emotionally and physically. It is the job of the physician to discuss as clearly as possible all the options available to the patient and all the potential risks and benefits of the paths they might choose. They must establish clear expectations as to what the pre and post-operative outcomes may look like. It is also important that the physician and institution of which they are apart work to provide all the resources that a patient may need to face all aspects of their care, even if it is simply additional time to process all that is happening.

The ramifications of the decisions these patients make extend throughout the remainder of their lives. The surgery that the patient undergoes will forever alter how their breast care will be provided, the ability of the breast care team to provide breast imaging, their breast exam, and their options for breast cancer surveillance. It is also worthy of reiterating that no surgery is without a risk of requiring additional surgery and this idea must be explored. The short term and long term complications of surgical intervention are significant as well and must be acknowledged, as should their risk for breast cancer development prior to surgery.

Beyond the immediately pre and postoperative changes noted after a patient undergoes breast reconstruction, the breast patient who undergoes mastectomy with reconstruction for breast cancer may necessitate some additional attention. The breast cancer survivor after mastectomy with reconstruction has increased physical and psychosocial needs related to treatment. Local treatments like radiation can increase the complication rates noted after reconstruction as well as increasing the risk of lymphedema associated with axillary surgery. Post-surgical range of motion may be an issue necessitating a physical therapy referral. Pain management may also need to be addressed.

The emotional component of breast cancer surgery should also be reemphasized as it is often under-appreciated and overlooked. Support groups, counseling services, psychological services should all be used as appropriate to ensure the mental health of the patient. Distress screening to evaluate for issues concerning to the patient should also be performed at regular intervals to ensure the patient's needs have not changed from prior discussions. Side effects related to systemic therapy should routinely be evaluated and treated as appropriate as they may have implications in regard to the emotional as well as physical components of their care.

Notably, in this setting surgical intervention does not only affect the individual it also can alter their relationships with others. The loss of a breast, no matter how cosmetically pleasing the outcome, alters the patient's self-image and with that their ability to feel like the whole and beautiful woman that they are. Their friends, family, and significant others are sure to see this in the way they relate to them; especially as far as moments of intimacy with their romantic partners. Relationship counseling or marriage counseling is an option that can be explored in this particular setting.

The surgical oncologist as well as the plastic surgeon and the remaining breast care team should strive to provide truly holistic care for their patients that takes all of the aforementioned points into consideration. All these concerns should be brought up and addressed at the earliest point possible to ensure the best physical and emotional outcome for the individual involved. Referrals should be made to appropriate team members if a patient's needs fall outside a particular area of expertise. The person as a whole must be incorporated into their care with their unique personality and goals of care taken into consideration; as it is only when we look at all aspects of an individual's needs that we can then provide the care that they deserve.

Acknowledgements

I would like to acknowledge and express my gratitude to all the mentors who contributed to my training and my patients who allowed me to care for them.

Conflict of interest

I have no conflicts of interest beyond the fact that my perspective may be biased as I am approaching this topic from the perspective of a breast surgical oncologist.

Author details

Karinn Chambers
ECU Health, Greenville, NC, USA

*Address all correspondence to: chambersk22@ecu.edu

IntechOpen

© 2023 The Author(s). Licensee IntechOpen. This chapter is distributed under the terms of the Creative Commons Attribution License (http://creativecommons.org/licenses/by/3.0), which permits unrestricted use, distribution, and reproduction in any medium, provided the original work is properly cited. (cc) BY

References

[1] American Society of Breast Surgeons. Position Statement on Screening Mammography. Available from: https://www.breastsurgeons.org/docs/statements/Position-Statement-on-Screening-Mammography.pdf [Accessed: May 5, 2023]

[2] National Comprehensive Cancer Network. NCCN Guidelines for Breast cancer Screening and Diagnosis. Version 2. 2013. Available from: http://www.nccn.org/professionals/physician_gls/f_guidelines.asp#breast_screening

[3] American Society of Plastic Surgeons. BIA-ALCL Summary. Available from: https://www.plasticsurgery.org/patient-safety/breast-implant-safety/bia-alcl-summary [Accessed: May 5, 2023]

[4] Bennett KG, Qi J, Kim HM, Hamill JB, Pusic AL, Wilkins EG. Comparison of 2-year complication rates among common techniques for postmastectomy breast reconstruction. JAMA Surgery. 2018;**153**(10):901-908. DOI: 10.1001/jamasurg.2018.1687

[5] Boughey JC, Attai DJ, et al. Contralateral prophylactic mastectomy consensus statement from the American Society of Breast Surgeons: Additional considerations and a framework for shared decision making. Annals of Surgical Oncology. 2016;**23**(10):3106-3111. DOI: 10.1245/s10434-016-5408-8

[6] Shaffer KM, Kennedy E, Glazer JV, Clayton AH, Cohn W, Millard TA, et al. Addressing sexual concerns of female breast cancer survivors and partners: A qualitative study of survivors, partners, and oncology providers about Internet intervention preferences. Support Care Cancer. 2021;**29**(12):7451-7460. DOI: 10.1007/s00520-021-06302-w

[7] Vegunta S, Kuhle CL, Vencill JA, Lucas PH, Mussallem DM. Sexual health after a breast cancer diagnosis: Addressing a forgotten aspect of survivorship. Journal of Clinical Medicine. 2022;**11**(22):6723. DOI: 10.3390/jcm11226723

Chapter 3

Immediate Breast Reconstruction with Implants

Evania Lok and Sally Ng

Abstract

Immediate breast reconstruction following mastectomy improves quality of life with benefits observed in body image and psychological health. An implant based reconstruction is one of the most common options utilised and a successful outcome relies on careful patient selection and technical decisions made intraoperatively. Significant technological adjuncts has advanced the role of direct to implant reconstruction by reducing rates of complications and implant failure. Understanding past techniques and variables in current practices facilitates operative management to provide an optimal implant based reconstructive outcome.

Keywords: breast reconstruction, breast implant, direct to implant, immediate breast reconstruction, mastectomy

1. Introduction

Historically, reconstructions post mastectomy was not widely adopted and the predominant options for women were mostly limited to simple acceptance of breast loss or use of an external prosthesis. The introduction of silicone breast implants in the 1960s heralded the modern breast reconstruction era. Implant based reconstruction is now one of the most utilised breast reconstructive techniques and has evolved from a two staged operation to a single stage procedure.

2. History of direct to implant reconstruction

Breast reconstruction has developed hand in hand with breast oncological resection.

The Halsted radical mastectomy was devised only 36 years after the introduction of anaesthesia [1]. For almost a century it reigned as the gold standard treatment for breast cancer. The resection was radical, involving total removal of breast tissue, full en bloc dissection of level 1–3 lymph nodes and pectoralis muscle [2]. The extensive surgery left patients with a concaved chest wall and minimal excess skin coverage. Contemporaneous reconstruction techniques mostly described surgeries to reconstruct the resultant skin defect utilising skin grafts or the Halsted technique of wound healing by secondary intention thought to be a deterrent for local recurrence [3]. In 1906 Tanzini sought a more robust option for skin coverage and was the first to describe a musculocutaneous flap in breast reconstruction by harvesting pedicled latissimus dorsi muscle and overlying skin [4]. The understanding of breast reconstruction in regard to the breast mound was first reported by Vincent Czerny in 1895 who transplanted a fist-sized lipoma from the patient's flank to their chest [5]. Similar attempts involving autologous tissue were described in the first half of the 20th Century with Ombredanne fashioning a new mound with pectoralis minor muscle while use of tubed pedicle flaps from the abdomen or gluteal tissue were pioneered by Gillies [6, 7]. None of these reconstructive options were widely adopted as they were lengthy multi-stage processes, expensive and associated with significant morbidity to donor and recipient sites. Advances in breast reconstruction were also limited during this time as Halsted believed it was a 'violation of the local control of disease' and actively discouraged the practice [3]. However in recent decades, breast cancer treatment has evolved towards breast conservation and ushered in modern reconstruction techniques ready to challenge traditional dogma.

The modern breast implant was developed by Cronin and Gerow in 1963 who recognised the resemblance of silicone gel within a plastic bag to a women's breast [8]. Initially adopted for cosmetic augmentation, Synderman and Guthrie first reported its use for breast reconstruction in 1971 [9]. They described a delayed procedure of minimum 6 months post radical mastectomy by careful sharp dissection of skin from chest wall. Symmetrising surgery could also be performed on the contralateral breast via either augmentation or reduction. Immediate breast reconstruction was initially avoided due to perceived compromise of oncological management and concern of negative psychological impact on a patient's body image. This was challenged by progressive reduction in the timing between resection and implant reconstruction until Noone et al. described a review of direct to implant surgeries [10]. This study demonstrated that direct to implant (DTI) reconstructions were safe operations which did not alter survival or recurrence rates nor impede adjunct treatments. Patient satisfaction with immediate reconstruction remained at a level consistent with delayed procedures and positively aided psychological acceptance of both mastectomy and aesthetic outcome.

Mastectomy practices similarly challenged the long established Halsted principles and less radical resections became accepted [11]. With the advent of skin and muscle sparing mastectomy, an opportunity arose for plastic surgeons to address issues with the subcutaneous implant reconstruction. Dissatisfactory appearance from capsular contraction and skin necrosis with subsequent risk to implant were both noted problems with often limited management options [12]. An immediate subpectoral implant reconstruction sought to remedy these concerns with an added benefit of providing additional soft tissue coverage to minimise the visible edge of an implant's superior ridge [13]. Despite this, DTI reconstructions were ultimately less adaptive to address concerns with implant position, size and shape and was subsequently supplanted by two stage tissue expansion/implant reconstruction and autologous techniques. However, the last two decades have witnessed a resurgence of DTI surgery in light of innovations which help to shape the breast pocket, optimally position the implant and assess mastectomy skin vascularity.

3. Role of direct to implant reconstruction

The DTI reconstruction offers immediate restoration of breast appearance as a single-stage approach performed at the time of mastectomy [14]. This avoids the prior technique of tissue expansion and subsequent exchange to implants. While eliminating the need for multiple episodes of tissue expansion and an inevitable secondary operation, it also negates the risk of additional postoperative complications and potential delay of adjuvant treatment. Significantly, DTI reconstructions are associated with a lack of donor site morbidity in comparison with autologous reconstruction resulting in a shorter recovery time and quicker return to work [14]. Considering the majority of breast cancers occur in the elderly population the appeal of a less invasive, single-stage procedure with prompt return to normal activities should not be overstated. Increased awareness and more rigorous screening have also led to an increase in younger women requiring oncological surgery [14]. Autologous reconstruction may be avoided in this cohort due to donor site morbidity despite improved cosmetic appearance. Timing or irradiation also plays a role in choosing between DTI and other forms of reconstruction. DTIs are associated with increased complications such as capsular contraction and implant extrusion particularly in the setting of irradiation when compared to autologous reconstruction [15]. However regardless of reconstruction type, any immediate reconstruction is associated with improved physical and psychological well being leading to decreased distress and anxiety associated with their cancer treatment [16].

Timing reconstructive surgery to occur concurrently with oncological resection has potential drawbacks. It requires coordination between two surgical teams which can delay surgery if schedules are not compatible. With different surgical teams, more theatre nurses are required to accommodate and theatre complexes may not be able to staff this easily. Ultimately combined surgery leads to a longer cumulative operative time and the potential for increased complications causing delays in adjuvant therapy. Immediate reconstruction also results in significantly less decision-making time for the patient and introduces the potential for the patient to lack a full understanding of reconstructive options and details of the procedure.

3.1 Psychosocial benefits

A diagnosis of breast cancer is a devastating and psychologically morbid experience for women of any age. Not only do concerns of oncological survival exist, but the physical impact of treatment should not be understated. Distress regarding breast disfigurement and loss of hair dominate, and the loss of these tenets of traditional femininity underscores feelings of unattractiveness and sexual disinterest following diagnosis [17]. Understandably anxiety and depression are also found in significant numbers in this cohort [17, 18]. Immediate reconstruction post-mastectomy can play a role in alleviating this psychosocial impact. Women who undergo immediate reconstruction score higher on measures of body image, sexuality and health-related quality of life particularly in comparison with women who underwent delayed reconstruction [19]. This may be reflective of less advanced disease seen in immediate reconstructive patients who may not even require additional adjuvant treatment. Certainly, the duration of delay is a significant contributor to psychological distress as immediate reconstruction patients were much less likely to recall post-operative distress than the delayed patients [20]. The overall decrease in distress is thought to arise from the fact that these patients do not experience loss of the breast mound and the psychological burden that loss entails. Regardless of reconstruction, anxiety and depression were uniformly improved for any reconstruction compared to mastectomy alone patients [19, 20]. The favourable psychosocial outcomes for immediate reconstruction should encourage all surgeons to make every effort for immediate reconstruction in suitable patients.

4. Preoperative considerations

4.1 Patient selection

Patient selection is a key consideration for DTI reconstruction. An ideal candidate would be a non-smoker with small to moderate breast size who desires to be a similar implant size [21]. Careful evaluation of their past medical and surgical history is recommended and physical assessment of the patient's features of weight, height, chest wall configuration and existing breast size and shape is essential. With any reconstructive surgery it is important to identify the aesthetic objective of the patient and to manage realistic expectations about the post operative breast. For patients seeking a significantly larger implant a two-stage expander to implant procedure may be more appropriate [22]. Breast characteristics of tissue laxity and resultant ptosis should prompt deliberation of concurrent mastopexy. Speculation of breast skin perfusion post mastectomy is required as scars, smoking and previous radiation can all affect mastectomy skin flap viability rendering DTI an unsuitable option. Conversely, in co-morbid patients who are not able to tolerate the operative burden of an autologous reconstruction, DTI may be the more appropriate surgery and careful patient evaluation is required in recommending the best reconstructive option [21, 22]. Communication with the patient is crucial to ensure they understand the long term ramifications of an implant reconstruction. Breast implants are not intended to last a lifetime and replacement, or removal is recommended 10–15 years after initial insertion [23]. This can be due to patient preference but most commonly due to long term sequelae of implants.

4.2 Implant selection

Choice of implant is an important component of DTI reconstruction and the goal for selection is to match the most appropriate implant to the patient. There exists multiple factors which contribute to an implant's success and each factor should be considered in relation to the individual. DTI reconstructions are often recommended for patients wishing to achieve a small to moderate implant size [24]. Larger implants can be associated with a higher rate of complications arising from increased tensile force on surgical wounds and increased pressure on mastectomy flaps contributing to tissue ischaemia. They may also result in less desired cosmetic outcomes of inferior displacement and over expansion of the lower pole [25]. The challenges of implant reconstruction following mastectomy compared to a purely cosmetic augmentation is the loss of glandular tissue and subsequent reduced soft tissue coverage which presents as upper pole hollowing and contour rippling. Implant shape affects how best to manage the post mastectomy breast cavity. Anatomical implants offer both superior and inferior pole projection resulting in the colloquial term "tear-drop implant". The ability to recreate a more natural appearing reconstructed breast has been suggested to reduce the need for subsequent symmetrising procedures on the contralateral breast.

However, the success of an anatomical implant relies on fixation of position which is difficult to maintain in the potential dead space following a mastectomy. The risks of malrotation can be mitigated with the use of a round implant which allows for more flexibility within the breast pocket [26–28]. Increasingly implant surface texture has been the pre-eminent focus on implant selection. Surface topography determines implant surface area and greater complexity of surface texture has a dramatic effect on cell-surface interactions and ultimately tissue integration [29]. This ability to determine tissue response resulted in highly textured implants which reduce risk of implant rotation and development of capsular contraction by adhering strongly to the breast pocket [30]. The trend of widespread textured implant use was abruptly albeit temporarily curtailed with the discovery of Breast Implant Associated Anaplastic Large Cell Lymphoma (BIA-ALCL) [31]. Though the advent of micro-textured implants theoretically adopts the advantages of the previous macro-textured implant without the BIA-ALCL risk, continued adoption of any textured implants over smooth implants remains controversial following oncological breast cancer surgery.

5. Intraoperative technique

Advances in breast cancer surveillance and treatment modalities have dramatically transformed the landscape of mastectomy techniques. Though radical mastectomy was the mainstay of treatment for decades, breast conservation surgery has emerged as the contemporary preference. Skin sparing mastectomy was first described in 1991 and consists of removal of all breast parenchyma and nipple areola complex (NAC) with removal of overlying skin of a superficially located neoplasm [32]. This technique maximally preserves skin to facilitate breast reconstruction. The NAC is integral to the perception of a naturally appearing breast and its loss is associated with worse patient psychosocial and sexual well-being. Efforts to retain the NAC led to the development of the nipple sparing mastectomy which sought to remove all breast parenchyma with total preservation of skin and NAC [33].

This evolution in breast surgery has allowed for greater adoption of DTI reconstruction as soft tissue viability of the breast pocket is retained. Sharp dissection in the plane between the subcutaneous tissue and breast parenchyma avoids ischaemic injury to the subdermal plexus of the mastectomy flaps. A multidisciplinary approach is required between the breast and plastic surgery teams to ensure adequate excision for oncological clearance is achieved while preserving the mastectomy skin flap vascularity to accommodate for DTI reconstruction [34]. Particularly as implant reconstruction historically fell out of favour in setting of high complication rates of wound dehiscence and implant extrusion, identifying tissue hypoperfusion can significantly alter the reconstructive plan. If any concerns are raised intraoperatively regarding skin perfusion the plastics team traditionally opted for a tissue expander and delayed implant reconstruction while waiting for any tissue necrosis to declare itself [35]. The use of indocyanine green angiography (ICG-A) has removed a lot of the guesswork by aiding assessment of skin perfusion and viability to minimise necrosis risk. ICG-A allows for real time visualisation of blood vessels up to 10 mm deep to the skin surface by intravenous injection of indocyanine green dye which binds to plasma proteins. Utilised in combination with imaging systems which can detect fluorescence produced by near-infrared light illumination of the dye, visual assessment of blood flow can be achieved [36]. This technology has advanced to hand held portable imaging devices which can be easily operated in theatre and its use in breast reconstruction has been proven to reduce rates of mastectomy flap necrosis [37].

Once adequate mastectomy skin flap viability has been established, pocket formation and implant position need to be defined. A pocket can derive from either the submuscular or subcutaneous plane. A submuscular pocket is formed by dissection of the relatively avascular plane deep to the pectoralis major muscle. An implant placed in this plane ensures additional soft tissue coverage over the implant and eliminates contact between the implant and skin incision. The extent of subpectoral dissection should be closely controlled to prevent both over and under sizing of the pocket. A wide pocket can cause implant displacement and rotation, while aggressive division of the inferior pectoralis major insertion can result in animation deformity. Aesthetically a muscular layer camouflages implant edges and minimises the appearance of rippling particularly in leaner patients but an underdeveloped pocket may compress the implant and create a more pronounced rippling effect. The pectoralis muscle would often not be adequate to completely cover the implant and recruiting either serratus anterior or rectus abdominis would be required to provide lower pole coverage [38]. Importantly a submuscular plane was shown to have the lowest incidence of capsular contraction when compared to other implant pocket positions [39].

A subcutaneous or pre pectoral approach was once the only available implant placement however they were fraught with complications in setting of more aggressive mastectomy techniques resulting in sub-optimal skin flaps. Soft tissue deficiencies increased the risk of extrusion, infection of the implants and capsular contraction was a common occurrence [40]. Understandably patients often chose to remove the implant and it was accepted that a subcutaneous DTI was not a recommended reconstructive option. Even with a better understanding of mastectomy skin vascularity and changes to mastectomy technique, the subcutaneous placement of an implant was still considered high risk and surgeons often chose a submuscular pocket as the safer plane [41]. Yet it was increasingly observed that the submuscular implant could not optimise aesthetic outcome. Complete muscular coverage of an implant would restrict lower pole expansion and was unable to mimic the appearance of a contralateral naturally ptotic breast. Efforts to address this problem resulted in surgeons releasing the inferior edge of the pectoralis muscle as a partial muscle or dual plane technique. Though this allowed for expansion of the lower pole of the breast, the loss of inferior fixation could result in the free edge of the muscle moving superiorly and compressing the surface of the implant creating a visible line when contracting.

5.1 Acellular dermal matrices and synthetic mesh

The invention of acellular dermal matrices (ADMs) and synthetic mesh provided surgeons the tools to adapt the breast pocket and optimise it for implant use. First introduced for breast reconstruction in 2005 [42], these surgical adjuncts have been widely adopted to improve implant position regardless of plane and offer additional support (**Figure 1**).

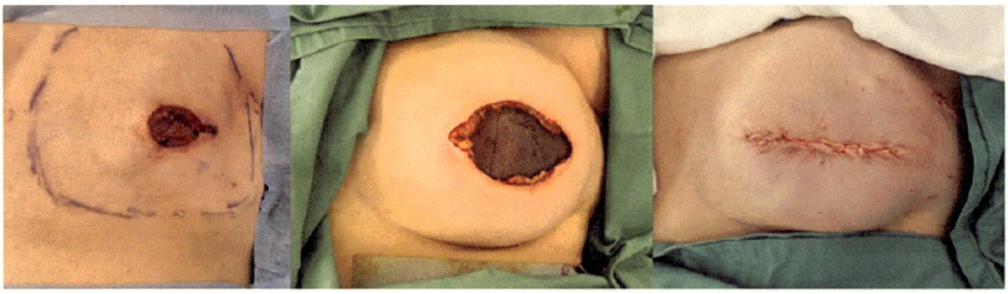

Figure 1.
Implant reconstruction following a skin sparing mastectomy. Robust mastectomy flaps envelope an implant with synthetic mesh support. The implant is inserted into the pre-pectoral plane and a tension free closure is achieved to primarily close the breast pocket.

ADMs are extracellular matrix structures which can be of either human, bovine or porcine origin. Processing removes cellular antigens which can elicit an immune response while preserving the structural matrix that encourages angiogenesis and tissue regeneration [43]. This lack of immunologic response allows for integration of the matrix to native tissue without encapsulation or contracture. ADMs are available as flat sheets of material that can be fashioned as required and many different applications of ADM have been described.

For submuscular implants, ADMs can artificially elongate the pectoralis muscle to cover the inferolateral pole of the implant which would be otherwise exposed in a dual-plane reconstruction negating the need to raise surrounding muscle for implant coverage [44]. Its use for pre pectoral implant placement has revolutionised this plane as a viable option for reconstruction. ADM can be formed as an internal bra surrounding the implant and securing it to the chest wall [45]. This can occur as anterior coverage only with the pectoralis major muscle in contact with the posterior surface of the implant. This technique masks upper pole implant visibility however it is technically more challenging to fashion the pocket without risking implant herniation or rotation. Complete coverage of the pre-pectoral implant requires a large volume of product to be secured together and aids in implant position. This provides an additional layer of tissue coverage and the additional support can relieve pressure on the mastectomy flaps. For both submuscular and prepectoral implants the use of ADM also helps to define and secure the inframammary fold while optimising implant position and lower pole projection [46].

Various synthetic meshes are also available on the market, providing an alternative to ADM. These meshes are incorporated through fibroblastic and foreign body reactions. They can be available as a preformed pocket thereby reducing surgical time when insetting and avoids over-handling of the product (**Figure 2**) [47]. ADMs have a significant economic burden and can be a deterrent to use while the relative cost-effectiveness of synthetic meshes makes it an appealing alternative option [48]. Meshes are also associated with less frequent infections and seroma formation in comparison with ADMs [49]. It is important to understand that though offering similar support, synthetic meshes do not provide additional soft tissue coverage, which ADMs can provide, and caution should be exercised with thin mastectomy skin flaps.

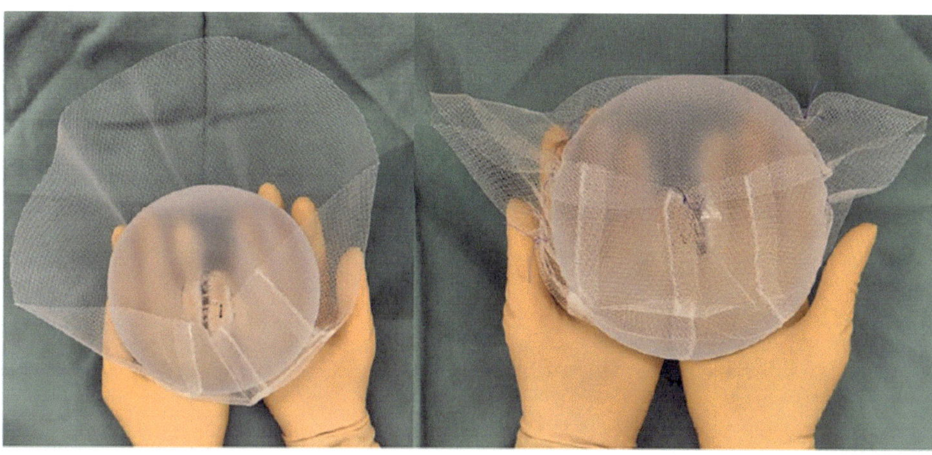

Figure 2.
The breast implant is placed within a synthetic mesh pocket. The mesh is sutured together to completely encompass the implant and to create fixation tabs from the excess material to enable optimal placement within the breast pocket.

6. Radiotherapy

Radiotherapy is an essential part of the multidisciplinary approach towards treating breast cancer. Post mastectomy radiotherapy is indicated with large tumour size (>5 cm), a positive margin, >4 positive lymph nodes on axillary dissection or cutaneous involvement. Early stage cancers with 1–3 positive nodes are also considered for treatment however hormone treatment is a reasonable alternative in older patients with stage 1 hormone receptor positive tumours. With the advent of neoadjuvant chemotherapy, radiotherapy is also recommended if the patient remains node positive post operatively [50]. These guidelines are derived from the substantial mortality benefit from postmastectomy radiotherapy and multidisciplinary discussion is recommended in their implementation. As early stage cancers are detected and treated earlier resulting in improved overall survival rates, the choice of reconstruction becomes increasingly important for long term quality of life. Radiotherapy has long been associated with soft tissue injury and inhibition of angiogenesis. It compromises breast pocket viability and wound healing while in the long term, irradiation of an implant based reconstruction can develop complications of capsular contraction and implant rupture [51]. Radiotherapy following implant reconstruction has consistently been associated with higher rates of reoperation and failure within the literature. Zhang et al. reported the reoperation rate as 15.4% compared to 6.7% of the control group while Chetta et al. observed that implants were 11 times more likely to result in reconstructive failure post radiotherapy relative to autologous reconstruction [52, 53]. The Mastectomy Reconstruction Outcomes Consortium (MROC) study, the most comprehensive review of post mastectomy radiation therapy, also found that major complications rates occurred in 33.2% of irradiated implant based reconstructions [54]. With this high incidence of complications, post mastectomy radiation is a relative contra-indication for DTI reconstruction.

7. Conclusion

Direct to implant is an excellent reconstructive option for patients who are suitable for immediate reconstruction and wanting to either maintain a similar or smaller breast volume. The use of acellular dermal matrix and synthetic mesh provides good lower pole support for the implant. Development of other adjuncts to assess mastectomy flap perfusion also aids in implant success and reduces rates of failure. Immediate breast reconstruction has noted advantages compared to a delayed approach and the use of implant reconstruction in this setting is dependent on appropriate patient selection and surgical technique.

Conflict of interest

The authors declare no conflict of interest.

Author details

Evania Lok and Sally Ng*
Austin Health, Victoria, Australia

*Address all correspondence to: sally.ng@austin.org.au

IntechOpen

© 2023 The Author(s). Licensee IntechOpen. This chapter is distributed under the terms of the Creative Commons Attribution License (http://creativecommons.org/licenses/by/3.0), which permits unrestricted use, distribution, and reproduction in any medium, provided the original work is properly cited.

References

[1] Halsted WS. The results of radical operations for the cure of carcinoma of the breast. Annals of Surgery. 1907;**46**(1):1-19

[2] Halsted WS. Developments in the skin-grafting operation for cancer of the breast. JAMA: The Journal of the American Medical Association. 1913;**60**(6):416

[3] Uroskie TW, Colen LB. History of breast reconstruction. Seminars in Plastic Surgery. 2004;**18**(2):65-69

[4] Tanzini I. Spora il mio nuova processo di amputazione della mammella. Riforma Medica. 1906;**22**(757)

[5] Czerny V. Plastic replacement of the breast with a lipoma (In German). Chir Kong Verhandl. 1895;**2**(2):216

[6] Teimourian B, Adham MN. Louis Ombredanne and the origin of muscle flap use for immediate breast mound reconstruction. Plastic and Reconstructive Surgery. 1983;**72**(6):905-910

[7] Gillies HD, Millard DR. Principles and Art of Plastic Surgery. Boston: Little Brown & Company; 1957

[8] Berry MG, Davies DM. Breast augmentation: Part I – A review of the silicone prosthesis. Journal of Plastic, Reconstructive & Aesthetic Surgery. 2010;**63**(11):1761-1768

[9] Snyderman RK, Guthrie RH. Reconstruction of the female breast following radical mastectomy. Plastic and Reconstructive Surgery. 1971;**47**(6):565-567

[10] Noone RB, Murphy JB, Spear SL, Little JW. A 6-year experience with immediate reconstruction after mastectomy for Cancer. Plastic and Reconstructive Surgery. 1985;**76**(2):258-269

[11] Cotlar AM, Dubose JJ, Michael RD. History of surgery for breast cancer: Radical to the sublime. Current Surgery. 2003;**60**(3):329-337

[12] Guthrie RH, Cucin RL. Breast reconstruction after mastectomy. Plastic and Reconstructive Surgery. 1980;**65**(5):595-602

[13] Salibian AA, Frey JD, Karp NS. Strategies and considerations in selecting between subpectoral and prepectoral breast reconstruction. Gland Surgery. 2019;**8**(1):11-18

[14] Perdanasari AT, Abu-Ghname A, Raj S, Winocour SJ, Largo RD. Update in direct-to-implant breast reconstruction. Seminars in Plastic Surgery. 2019;**33**(04): 264-269

[15] Zugasti A, Hontanilla B. The impact of adjuvant radiotherapy on immediate implant-based breast reconstruction surgical and satisfaction outcomes: A systematic review and Meta-analysis. Plastic and Reconstructive Surgery – Global Open. 2021;**9**(11):e3910

[16] Heimes AS, Stewen K, Hasenburg A. Psychosocial aspects of immediate versus delayed breast reconstruction. Breast Care. 2017;**12**(6):374-377

[17] Schover LR. The impact of breast cancer on sexuality, body image, and intimate relationships. CA: A Cancer Journal for Clinicians. 1991;**41**(2):112-120

[18] Puigpinós-Riera R, Graells-Sans A, Serral G, Continente X, Bargalló X,

Domènech M, et al. Anxiety and depression in women with breast cancer: Social and clinical determinants and influence of the social network and social support (DAMA cohort). Cancer Epidemiology. 2018;**55**:123-129

[19] Stevens LA, McGrath MH, Druss RG, Kister SJ, Gump FE, Forde KA. The psychological impact of immediate breast reconstruction for women with early breast cancer. Plastic and Reconstructive Surgery. 1984;**73**(4):619-626

[20] Dean C, Chetty U, Forrest APM. Effects of immedicate breast reconstruction of psychosocial morbidity after mastectoy. The Lancet. 1983;**321**(8322):459-462

[21] Cassileth L, Kohanzadeh S, Amersi F. One-stage immediate breast reconstruction with implants. Annals of Plastic Surgery. 2012;**69**(2):134-138

[22] Salzberg CA. Direct-to-implant breast reconstruction. Clinics in Plastic Surgery. 2012;**39**(2):119-126

[23] Lieffering AS, Hommes JE, Ramerman L, Rakhorst HA, Mureau MAM, Verheij RA, et al. Prevalence of local postoperative complications and breast implant illness in women with breast implants. JAMA Network Open. 2022;**5**(10):e2236519

[24] Scuderi N, Alfano C, et al. Multicenter study on breast reconstruction outcome using ecker implants. Aesthetic Plastic Surgery. 2010;**35**(1):66-72

[25] Medor MC, Bouhadana G, Churchill IF, Hemmerling T, Bonapace-Potvin M, Papanastasiou C, et al. How big is too big? Exploring the relationship between breast implant volume and postoperative complication rates in primary breast augmentations. Plastic and Reconstructive Surgery – Global Open. 2023;**11**(3):e4843

[26] Khavanin N, Clemens MW, Pusic AL, Fine NA, Hamill JB, Kim HM, et al. Shaped versus round implants in breast reconstruction. Plastic and Reconstructive Surgery. 2017;**139**(5):1063-1070

[27] Gardani M, Bertozzi N, et al. Breast reconstruction with anatomical implants: A review of indications and techniques based on current literature. Annals of Medicine and Surgery. 2017;**21**:96-104

[28] Stevens WG, Harrington J, Alizadeh K, Broadway D, Zeidler K, Godinez TB. Eight-Year Follow-Up Data from the U.S. Clinical Trial for Sientra's FDA-approved round and shaped implants with high-strength cohesive silicone gel. Aesthetic Surgery Journal. 2015;**35**(suppl_1):S3-S10

[29] Doloff JC, Veiseh O, de Mezerville R, Sforza M, Perry TA, Haupt J, et al. The surface topography of silicone breast implants mediates the foreign body response in mice, rabbits and humans. Nature Biomedical Engineering. 2021;**5**(10):1115-1130

[30] Maxwell GP, Scheflan M, Spear S, Nava MB, Hedén P. Benefits and limitations of macrotextured breast implants and consensus recommendations for optimizing their effectiveness. Aesthetic Surgery Journal. 2014;**34**(6):876-881

[31] McKernan C. Treating breast implant-associated anaplastic large cell lymphoma. JAAPA. 2021;**34**(4):47-51

[32] Toth BA, Lappert P. Modified skin incisions for mastectomy. Plastic and Reconstructive Surgery. 1991;**87**(6):1048-1053

[33] Ashikari AY, Kelemen PR, Tastan B, Salzberg CA, Ashikari RH. Nipple sparing mastectomy techniques: A literature review and an inframammary technique. Gland Surgery. 2018;**7**(3): 273-287

[34] Bertozzi N, Pesce M, Santi P, Raposio E. One-stage immediate breast reconstruction: A concise review. BioMed Research International. 2017;**2017**:1-12

[35] Pusic AL, Cordeiro PG. Breast reconstruction with tissue expanders and implants: A practical guide to immediate and delayed reconstruction. Seminars in Plastic Surgery. 2004;**18**(2):71-77

[36] Driessen C, Arnardottir TH, Lorenzo AR, Mani MR. How should indocyanine green dye angiography be assessed to best predict mastectomy skin flap necrosis? A systematic review. Journal of Plastic, Reconstructive & Aesthetic Surgery. 2020;**73**(6):1031-1042

[37] Lauritzen E, Bredgaard R, Bonde C, Jensen LT, Damsgaard TE. Indocyanine green angiography in breast reconstruction: A narrative review. Annals of Breast Surgery. 2022;**6**:6-6

[38] Hwang DY, Park SH, Kim SW. A modified dual-plane technique using the serratus anterior fascia in primary breast augmentation. Plastic and Reconstructive Surgery Global Open. 2017;**5**(2):e1213-e1213

[39] Headon H, Kasem A, Mokbel K. Capsular contracture after breast augmentation: An update for clinical practice. Archives of Plastic Surgery. 2015;**42**(5):532

[40] Gruber RP, Kahn R, Lash H, Maser MR, Apfelberg DB, Laub DR. Breast reconstruction following mastectomy. Plastic and Reconstructive Surgery. 1981;**67**(3):312-317

[41] Schlenker JD, Bueno RA, Ricketson G, Lynch JB. Loss of silicone implants after subcutaneous mastectomy and reconstruction. Plastic and Reconstructive Surgery. 1978;**62**(6):853-861

[42] Breuing KH, Warren SM. Immediate bilateral breast reconstruction with implants and inferolateral AlloDerm slings. Annals of Plastic Surgery. 2005;**55**(3):232-239

[43] Badylak S, Freytes D, Gilbert T. Extracellular matrix as a biological scaffold material: Structure and function. Acta Biomaterialia. 2009;**5**(1):1-13

[44] Ganske I, Verma K, Rosen H, Eriksson E, Chun YS. Minimizing complications with the use of acellular dermal matrix for immediate implant-based breast reconstruction. Annals of Plastic Surgery. 2013;**71**(5):464-470

[45] Breuing KH, Colwell AS. Inferolateral AlloDerm hammock for implant coverage in breast reconstruction. Annals of Plastic Surgery. 2007;**59**(3):250-255

[46] Macadam SA, Lennox PA. Acellular dermal matrices: Use in reconstructive and aesthetic breast surgery. Canadian Journal of Plastic Surgery. 2012;**20**(2):75-89

[47] Faulkner HR, Shikowitz-Behr L, McLeod M, Wright E, Hulsen J, Austen WG. The use of absorbable mesh in implant-based breast reconstruction: A 7-year review. Plastic & Reconstructive Surgery. 2020;**146**(6):731e-736e

[48] Jose F, Moraes R. Synthetic mesh as a potential low-cost alternative to dermal matrix in mammary reconstructions. Revista Brasileira de Cirurgia Plástica. 2021;**36**(2):122-128

[49] Choi YS, Deok-Woo DW, You HJ, Lee TY. Comparing complications of biologic and synthetic mesh in breast reconstruction: A systematic review and network meta-analysis. Archives of Plastic Surgery. 2022;**50**(1):3-9

[50] EBCTCG (Early Breast Cancer Trialists' Collaborative Group). Effect of radiotherapy after mastectomy and axillary surgery on 10-year recurrence and 20-year breast cancer mortality: meta-analysis of individual patient data for 8135 women in 22 randomised trials. The Lancet. 2014;**383**(9935):2127-2135

[51] Anderson JF, Hammond JB, Thorpe CS, Kosiorek HE, Pockaj BA, Gray RJ, et al. Capsular contracture after radiation therapy following mastectomy and implant-based reconstruction. International Journal of Radiation Oncology Biology Physics. 2019;**105**(1):E50-0

[52] Zhang L, Jin K, Wang X, Yang Z, Wang J, Ma J, et al. The impact of radiotherapy on reoperation rates in patients undergoing mastectomy and breast reconstruction. Annals of Surgical Oncology. 2019;**26**(4):961-968

[53] Chetta MD, Aliu O, Zhong L, Sears ED, Waljee JF, Chung KC, et al. Reconstruction of the irradiated breast. Plastic and Reconstructive Surgery. 2017;**139**(4):783-792

[54] Wilkins EG, Hamill JB, Kim HM, Kim JY, Greco RJ, Qi J, et al. Complications in Postmastectomy breast reconstruction. Annals of Surgery. 2018;**267**(1):164-170

Chapter 4

Direct-to-Implant Breast Reconstruction Method: Muscle Anchoring Technique Using Absorbable Strings and Its Safety

Naoki Watanabe, Shoko Otsuka, Sena Hori, Haruyuki Takata and Takeshi Yuasa

Abstract

In prosthesis-based breast reconstruction, surgeons select the sub-muscle layer for implant placement, but the pectoralis major muscle is not sufficient to cover the implant. The pectoralis major muscle does not reach the inframammary sulcus line, so the muscle pockets for implant inevitably have defects. From 2016 to 2019, we performed direct-to-implant (DTI) breast reconstruction for 123 patients, during which the implant was placed partially under the muscle plane and the inferior-lateral portion was placed directly underneath the skin flap. We divided the pectoralis major muscle and serratus anterior muscle in their origin partially and arranged their shape and position. To maintain their intended placement, we used the absorbable mesh sling. From 2020, we had arranged this method and performed DTI in 35 patients using absorbable strings simply as a substitute for mesh. The DTI reconstruction using mesh or using absorbable strings could show the acceptable safety and feasibility. Both techniques were associated with a low risk of surgical complications, reoperation (with mesh 4.1%, and without mesh 0%), and removal of implant (with mesh 2.4%, and without mesh 0%).

Keywords: direct-to-implant, breast reconstruction, early surgical complication, absorbable mesh sling, anchoring by absorbable strings

1. Introduction

In Japan, allograft skin is not covered by public health insurance and cannot be used for breast reconstruction in practice. In such a situation, we have pursued the optimal methodology of direct-to-implant (DTI) breast reconstruction with various ideas [1, 2]. Since 2019, we have started a new method and have obtained good outcomes, so I would like to report it here.

2. Muscle anchoring technique using absorbable strings

2.1 Anatomical constraints in breast reconstruction using implant

Of the prosthesis-based reconstructive surgeries that are performed at the same time as radical surgery for breast cancer, the process can be classified into two.

One is direct-to-implant (DTI) reconstruction, in which the space created by resection of mammary tissue is replaced immediately with an implant as it is. Then the reconstruction process is completed at the same time as breast cancer surgery. This procedure does not force the patient to experience breast loss. The other is to temporarily place a tissue expander in the space after resection, and gradually expand it after the wound heal. It is to stretch the chest skin and the surrounding muscles that cover the tissue expander. After obtaining sufficient space for the implant, the tissue expander is replaced with an appropriate implant at the right time. The patients will have to undergo two surgeries (two-stage reconstruction).

The mammary gland is completely removed by nipple-sparing mastectomy (NSM) or skin-sparing mastectomy (SSM), and almost all of the breast skin is preserved in both surgeries. Therefore, it is not necessary to stretch the mammary gland skin primarily. Then why is two-stage process needed after NSM and SSM?

This is because the pectoralis major muscle does not have sufficient area to cover the implant. Both length and width are insufficient (**Figure 1** left). The skin-flap in the lower half area of the breast mound bears the weight of the implant. Because the pectoralis major muscle does not reach that far, the skin bears the implant independently. Certainly, if the surrounding muscles such as the serratus anterior, rectus abdominis, transversus abdominis, and anterior oblique muscles are all mobilized, we could make a complete pocket with the muscles (**Figure 1** right). If you go that far, however, it would be wiser to reconstruct the mammary glands with only muscles. Therefore, in two-stage breast reconstruction, a tissue expander was once inserted, a

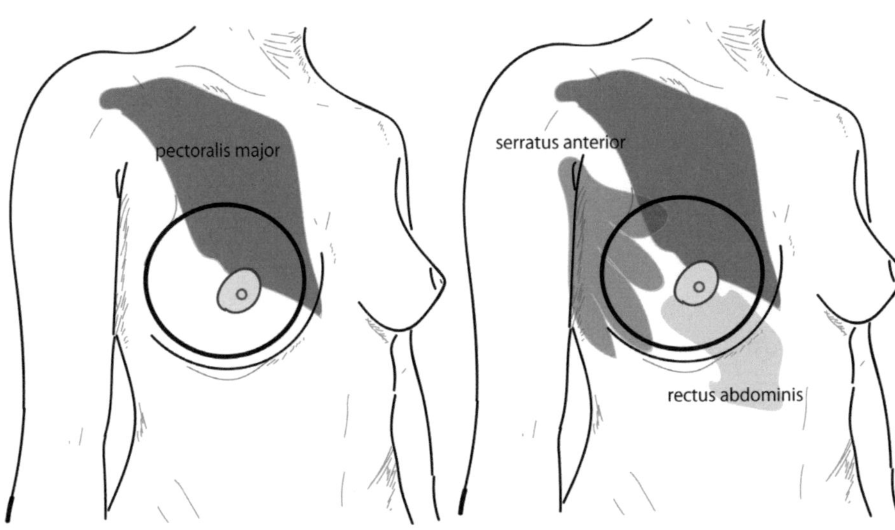

Figure 1.
The pectoralis major muscle does not have a sufficient area to anatomically cover the surface of the implant, and a sizable portion of the surrounding muscles would need to be sacrificed to adequately conceal the entire implant.

capsule was created with the pectoralis major muscle and, in some cases, a part of the serratus anterior muscle, and the muscle was stretched over time.

To solve this anatomical problem, in the United States, Alloderm® (Allergan U.S.A. K.K.) is applied as a patch to reinforce the areas that cannot be covered with the pectoralis major muscle. Alloderm® is a commercially available medical material that can be applied to anyone by treating the dermis of the skin collected from a donor's body to inactivate antigenicity. Alloderm® is sure that it could patch and reinforce the lower area of breast mound, but it has no blood flow and no immune function that protects from bacterial infection. Since Alloderm® is premised on a body donation so it is not covered by public health insurance in Japan.

2.2 Direct-to-implant reconstruction that can be implemented in Japan

In 2016, Tessler et al. first reported a method of using VICRYL mesh® (Ethicon, Johnson & Johnson K.K., JAPAN) instead of Alloderm® to connect the pectoralis major muscle and the chest wall to cover the inferior area that cannot be patched by the pectoralis major muscle alone [3]. Unlike Alloderm®, VICRYL mesh® is an absorbable material. It has a temporary reinforcing effect on the flap in the inferior area, but it will continue for 2 weeks, just like VICRYL PLUS® absorbable strings. After absorption, it lost its function. However, they reported the excellent outcomes of their absorbable mesh-sling procedure; 2.6% of cases had flap necrosis, 1.3% had infection, 1.3% required revision surgery due to implant displacement, and only 1.3% had implant removal. We have adopted this procedure since 2016 and have performed it in 123 cases to date.

Faulkner et al. used this technique to perform 227 reconstructions in 227 cases and reported the results of 7 years of observation [4]. As a matter to be noticed, they performed postoperative radiotherapy in 20.5% of cases. As a result, they also showed good results; flap necrosis (requiring invasive procedure) was 3.5%, infection was 2.1%, and implant removal was 4.5%.

Tessler does not use the serratus anterior muscle, only the pectoralis major muscle serves its purpose. Therefore, the only role of the absorbable VICRYL Mesh® is to place the pectoralis major muscle in a caudal stretched state as much as possible and to wait for the adhesion between the pectralis major muscle and the skin flap at the appropriate position intended by the surgeon. Using this absorbable mesh-sling method, then we could perform DTI reconstruction surgery even in Japan, where Alloderm® cannot be used.

2.3 Arrange and place the muscle body and implants appropriately

Figure 2 shows our method, which is a modification of Tessler's one, currently in use. The pectoralis major muscle and the serratus anterior muscle are arranged and placed properly to cover the implant, by using absorbable strings like shoelaces. Unlike Tessler, our new method does not use mesh on the purpose. In practice, VICRYL PLUS 4–0® ("4–0" is a USP size and the diameter of the string is 0.2 mm.) is used, but these "shoelaces" are used to make tension and anchor between the muscle and the subcutaneous area of the inframammary sulcus. The pectoralis major muscle is partially dissected at its origin and is separated as needed. The top of the mammary gland mound, around the areola, has the least blood flow. There should be support from underneath with the pectoralis major muscle as much as possible. The serratus anterior can also be mobilized as needed simultaneously. In this case, it is not

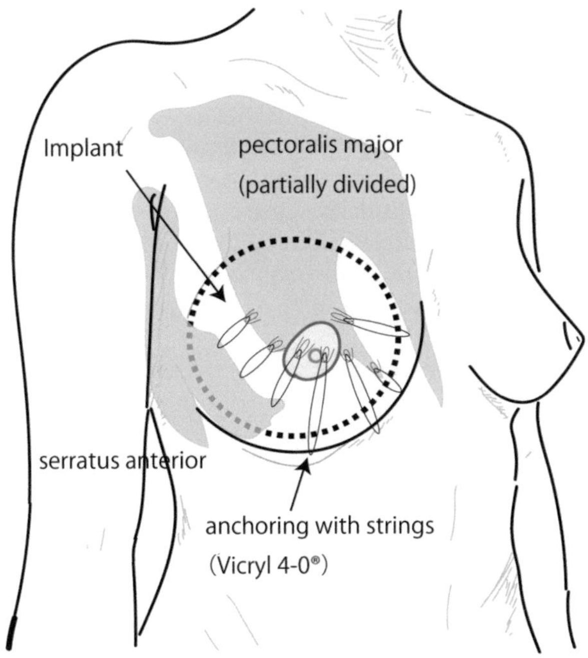

Figure 2.
The pectoralis major muscle and the serratus anterior muscle are arranged and placed properly to cover the implant, by using absorbable strings as if like shoelaces. VICRYL PLUS 4–0® is used to make tension and anchor between the muscle and the subcutaneous area of the inframammary sulcus.

necessary to dissect the origin of the muscle body in its entire length. It is possible for the fascia of serratus anterior muscle alone to serve its purpose (**Figure 3**).

With this method, the pectoralis major muscle can be moved to the desired position. Whether the surgery is SSM or NSM with a peri-areolar incision, around the incision is with the highest risk of ischemic skin necrosis. With the mobilization of the pectoralis major muscle, it is possible to support the suture directly from underneath by the muscle body with rich blood microcirculation (**Figure 3**). The papilla, which is prone to ischemia, can also be supported. In a case, if the sub-mammary sulcus is incised, it can be supported from underneath with part of the serratus anterior muscle. Even if the required implant weight is heavy, it can be supported from below by not only skin flap but the serratus anterior muscle. If the surgeon needs the appearance of breast ptosis, surgeons should also consider not using the serratus anterior.

Since 2020, at our facility, we have performed DTI reconstruction in 35 cases using this anchoring technique with absorbable strings. We will retrospectively examine the results and the risk of complications in a group of patients who underwent DTI reconstruction using this technique (without Mesh) and compare them with 123 patients who underwent DTI using the Tessler method (with Mesh).

2.4 Surgical technique

The operations are performed under general anesthesia. At the start, we perform ultrasonography to confirm the location of tumor. To avoid the tumor contamination

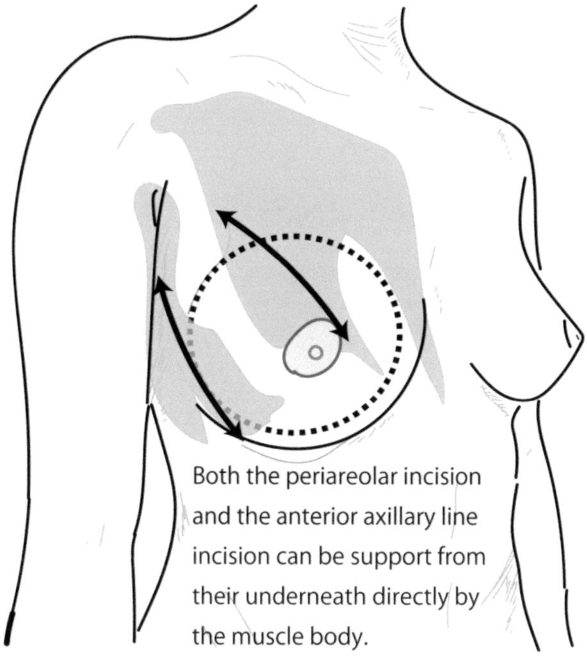

Figure 3.
Even minimal ischemic necrosis at the wound edge can also cause infection. The underlayer of the incision is completely covered by the muscle tissue.

in the flap, we put a mark at the point where the tumor should edge up to the skin by injecting the pigment. During the operation, we harvested the subcutaneous tissue from the flap side and submitted to the immediate pathological examination.

On a case-by-case basis, sentinel lymph node biopsy or axillary lymph node dissection will be performed. Surgery to the axilla should not influent the indication for, or the procedure of breast reconstruction, aside from skin incision. The surgeon has to choose whether skin incision the inframammary line or the line around the nipple-areolar circle and extending to the axilla. In the case requiring the axillar dissection, we routinely select the later incision.

First, it is important to find the superficial layer of superficial fascia in the incision, then we start exfoliation of mammary glands from the skin in appropriate layers. After reaching underneath the nipple, we get the sample of the specimen and provide to the intraoperative pathological examination by frozen section. If the malignant involvement was recognized, we convert the NSM, even if you planned, into SSM with the nipple-areolar complex resection. Similarly, the malignant involvement at the site above the tumor should be coped with widening the skin resection enough and properly. If the area of flap got too tighter to cover the desired implant, we should convert DTI into two-stage using the proper tissue expander.

After completion of skin-preserving mastectomy, we start reconstruction by creating appropriate subpectoral pocket. We release the pectoralis major muscle at its origin on the sternum, if it was right breast, proceeded to the 3- and 9- o'clock levels. Occasionally, we add the slitting the pectoralis along the muscle bundles and adjusted its position (**Figure 4**).

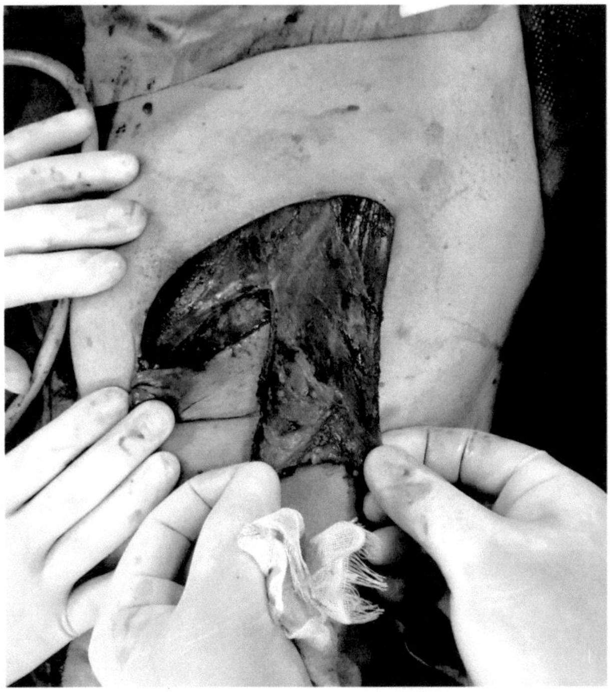

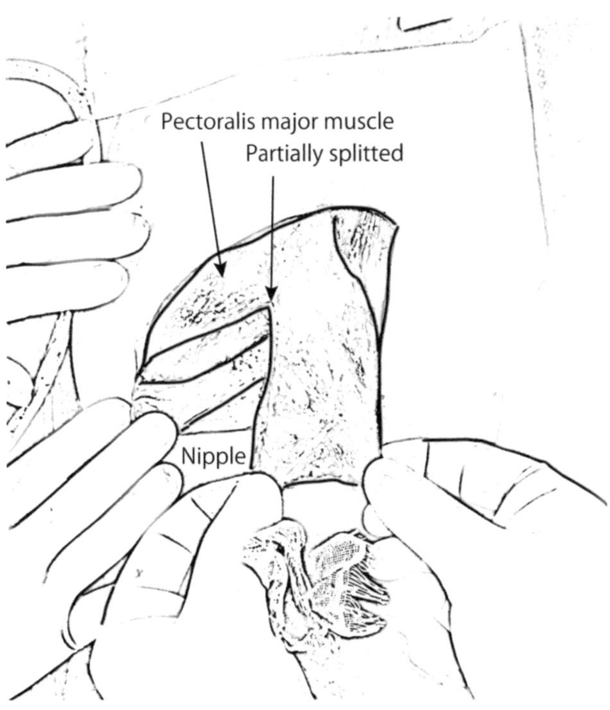

Figure 4.
The pectoralis major muscle was partially released from its origin on the sternum. If it was the right breast, the release extended to the 3- and 9-o'clock levels. Occasionally, we also make a slit in the pectoralis along the muscle bundle.

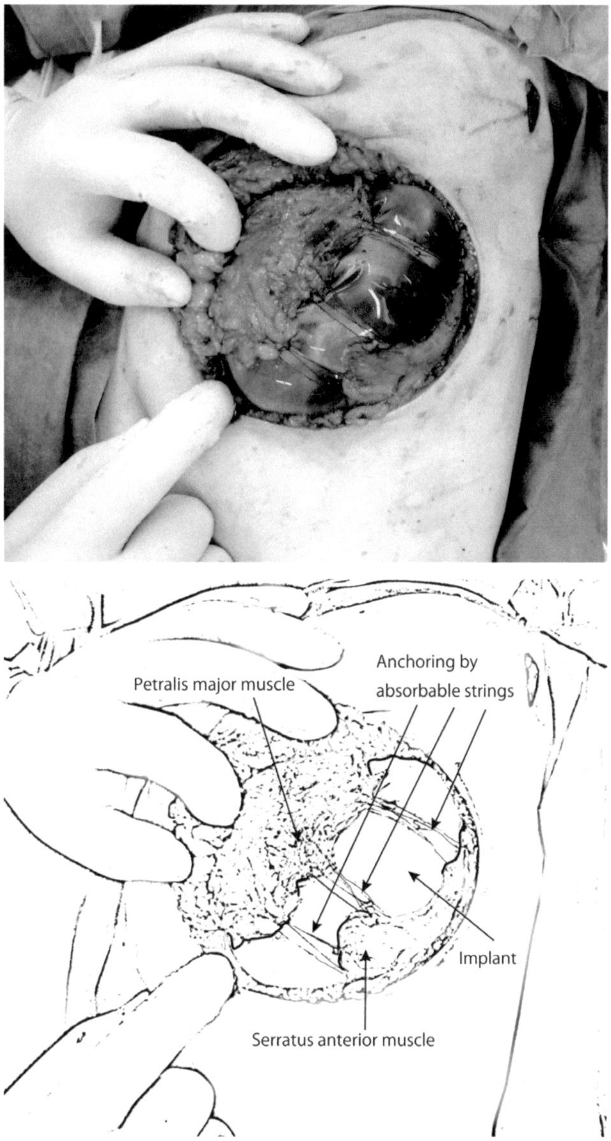

Figure 5.
After placement of the implant, we start suturing between the pectoralis major muscle and lateral and inferior fold, or between the pectoralis major muscle and the fascia of serratus anterior muscle, using the absorbable string (VICRYL PLUS® 4–0). We refrain from using mesh to anchor the muscle body to the needed site.

A saline sizer was placed in the subpectoral pocket and inflated to the desired volume. While checking the appearance of the mammary gland, we select the best cohesive according to the size of the sizer and the weight of the removed breast weight.

We decide whether to use the serratus anterior fascia at this time. If the width of the pectoralis major muscle defect covering the implant is likely to exceed 4 cm, it should be used in combination. There are demerits due to detachment and use of the serratus anterior fascia; increased postoperative pain, and loss of breast ptotic appearance.

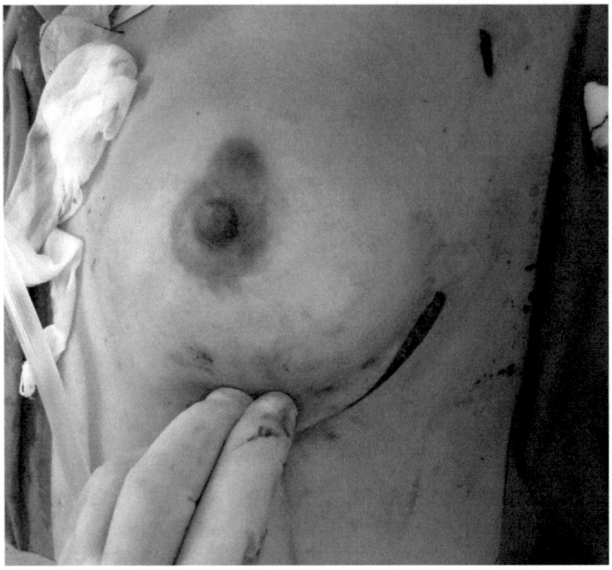

Figure 6.
The photograph depicts a stage where the surgery is nearly finished, and only the skin remains to be sutured.

After placement of the appropriate implant in the pocket, we start suturing between the pectoralis major muscle and lateral and inferior fold, or between the pectoralis major muscle and the fascia of serratus anterior muscle, using the absorbable string (VICRYL PLUS® 4–0). The important thing here is not to overtighten the string to the end (**Figure 5**). We believe that we should not tighten the thread, just like we do with shoelaces. We just keep in mind that it is enough if there is a muscle body under the incision.

Then, suction drains were placed. Adjustments were made as necessary, hemostasis was ensured, and the wound was then closed (**Figure 6**).

3. Assessment of complications

In the Tessler method, between the pectoralis major muscle and a part of the serratus anterior muscle or inframammary sulcus line are slung using an absorbable mesh (VICRYL Mesh®). From 2016 to the present, we performed the DTI breast reconstruction in 123 patients (with mesh). In December 2019, we started to apply our modified method in which the pectoralis major muscle and inframammary sulcus are anchored using only absorbable strings (VICRYL PLUS® 4–0) like shoelaces without using absorbable mesh. Thirty-five patients underwent DTI reconstruction with this method (Without Mesh).

Although both VICRYL Mesh® and VICRYL PLUS® 4–0 are absorbable substances, it is a foreign substance. If the amount of the use is reduced, it is expected that surgical site infections will also decrease.

We retrospectively compared the outcome, especially from the viewpoint of complication due to ischemia in 35 patients who underwent DTI without Mesh and 123 patients with Mesh.

To check for surgical complications, we checked ischemic changes and surgical site infections for all patients during hospitalization, and in visiting the hospital as an outpatient about 1 and 2 weeks after surgery. Since 2010, we have been prospectively investigating complications in breast reconstruction cases at our institution. We checked and made an independent database for the occurrence and time of occurrence (days after surgery) about the following items; presence of seroma, wound edge necrosis, nipple ischemia or necrosis, surgical site infection (SSI), hematoma formation, hospitalization due to complications, request of reoperation due to complications, and implant removal. Other complications are described and evaluated.

In this study, we did the assessment in using this database, but hence, we did not consider implant displacement, the presence or absence of capsular contracture, deformation, which should be accessed in long-term observation. The grade classification of complications was based on Common Terminology Criteria for Adverse Events (CTCAE) Version 5.0 Published: Nov 27, 2017 and Japanese translation by JCOG [5].

Because we examined perioperative complications observed within 2 months after surgery, postoperative adjuvant treatments such as chemotherapy, radiotherapy, and hormone agents are, if any, almost negligible. We have never performed bilateral simultaneous DTI breast reconstruction.

For statistical analysis, the computer software EZR was used [6]. The analysis method was described for each.

3.1 Result

Since this study is a retrospective analysis, it is not appropriate to compare significant differences in complication rates in two methods (with or without Mesh).

First, the time when the surgery was performed was different, so the learning curve of the operator affected against the group without mesh (**Table 1**). Second, some significant differences are shown in the patient background; in the presence or absence of hypertension as a medical history, T factor, and stage in the TNM classification. With mesh group, which includes more advanced cases, is at a disadvantage. On the other side, without mesh group underwent a larger mastectomy and was reconstructed using a larger implant. In this regard, without mesh group is at a significant disadvantage (**Table 1**).

Complications occurred from the day of surgery to 43 days. We experienced cases of surgical site infection (SSI) on the 137th day and the 202nd day in the with mesh group. These were not perioperative complications, but due to a local trauma. Excluding these, the mean time to SSI was 12.5 days.

Overall complications were not affected by the presence or absence of Mesh, and indeed no significant difference was observed. We expected a decrease in SSI by not using mesh, but this was not observed. Concerning about any ischemic changes around the wound, we checked even small ones, which patients do not seem to notice, and converted them into data according to the grade. However, no increase was observed even after stopping the use of Mesh (**Table 2**).

Through the recruitment period, only three cases in the with mesh group resulted in discontinuation of reconstruction with IMP removal.

	With Mesh (n = 123)	Without Mesh (n = 35)	
Age (years)	45.8 ± 6.1 (22–63)	45.3 ± 4.2 (35–56)	p = 0.677¶
Body-mass index (kg/m^2)	21.5 ± 3.0 (16.83–32.7)	22.3 ± 2.6 (18.03–27.61)	p = 0.166¶
DM(−/+)	119/1 Uncertain 3	35/0	p = 1.0§
HT(−/+)	120/3	34/1	P<0.001§
Smoking (Never/ Quit[*1])	110/11 Uncertain 2	30/5	p = 0.357§
Neoadjuvant chemotherapy (−/+)	110/13	31/4	p = 0.519§
T[*2] (is/ 1/ 2/ 3/ 4)	(50/ 50/ 15/ 7/ 1)	(19/ 11 /5 /0 /0)	p = 0.00052
Stage[*3] (0 /1 /2 /3 /4)	(51/ 46/ 18/ 7/ 0)	(19 /6 /5 /1 /1)	P < 0.001
Surgery			
Operation time (min)	125.5 ± 22.9 (78.0–186.0)	128.4 ± 23.4 (60.0–175.0)	p = 0.520¶
Bleeding (ml)	91.9 ± 65.5 (nearly 0–410)	86.7 ± 59.3 (nearly 0–260)	p = 0.680¶
Mastectomy weight (g)[*4]	211.2 ± 119.9 (130–567)	277.0 ± 114.4 (54–552)	p = 0.00493¶
Implant Volume (ml)	229.0 ± 89.9 (170–595)	294.1 ± 65.6 (190–415)	p = 0.00463¶
NSM/SSM	117/6	32/3	p = 0.416§
Ax (0-SLNB/ I-II)	103/20	28/7	p = 0.615§

**1 Smokers were instructed to abstain from smoking for at least 28 days before surgery.*
**2 We took the value of cT at admission as the value of pT, in the case of requiring neoadjuvant chemotherapy.*
**3 We took the value of cStage at admission as the value of pStage, in the case of requiring neoadjuvant chemotherapy.*
**4 Including cases in which margins were positive in the first surgery and subcutaneous mastectomy was performed in reoperation.*
¶Student-t.
§Fisher's Exact Test χ^2 test.

Table 1.
Baseline characteristics.

	With Mesh (n = 123)		Without Mesh (n = 35)		
	Grade 1–2	Grade 3	Grade 1–2	Grade 3	
Seroma	4 (3.3%)	0	0	0	p = 0.576§
Ischemic change (in nipple, areola, wound area)	19 (15.4%)	0	4 (11.4%)	1 (2.9%)	p = 0.786§
Surgical site infection	5 (4.1%)	5 (4.1%)	1 (2.6%)	0	P = 1§
Hematoma	4 (3.3%)	0	3 (8.6%)	0	p = 0.183§
Hospitalization due to complications	7 (5.7%)		1 (2.9%)		p = 0.686§
Request of reoperation due to complications,	5 (4.1%)		0		p = 0.588§
Implant removal	3 (2.4%)		0		p = 1§

§Fisher's Exact Test χ^2 test.

Table 2.
Adverse events per breast.

4. Discussion

4.1 Anchoring with absorbable materials

Our series with absorbable mesh sling or with absorbable anchor strings for DTI breast reconstruction confirmed Tessler's excellent results with a low complication profile [3]. As well as their experience, the complications in our series were more favorable than that reported complication profiles of up to 14.8–18% for DTI with using Allodermnew® [7, 8] and 33.9% of reoperation incidence, and 10.9% of explantation and replacement in the Mentor [9] study. Our results are encouraging for Japanese surgeons, who cannot access Alloderm® at present. Both Vicryl mesh® and Vicryl PLUS® are widely available and relatively inexpensive materials, which have been used in numerous surgical procedures for many years.

We experienced surgical site infection (Grade 1–2) in this series (4.1% in group with mesh, 2.6% in group without mesh). In one case of them, we had misled the inadequate candidate who was with atopic active dermatitis to the implant-based reconstruction. Through these experiences, we found thought-provoking facts concerning about the infectious complication in using the implant that surgical site infection could develop in outpatients even more than 6 weeks after the surgery. From these findings, we made a hypothesis that these infections were not usual surgical site infections, and might be caused by the lymphogenous dissemination of "hand or finger contamination" from the patients' everyday affairs. We now routinely give the patients specific guidance on hand hygiene; occasionally glove use to steer clear of injury, daily skin care, and avoidance of gardening or handling of kitchen garbage. We keep them strictly in order, especially during the three months after the surgery. SSI complications were obviously reduced since we started this guidance.

As this fact shows, patient cooperation is essential for successful reconstructive surgery. Smoking cessation in the perioperative period would be an almost absolute requirement.

Implant exposure is the major complication requiring the explantation. To prevent this tragedy, it is important to cover of the implant with the healthy muscle to the extent possible. Although complete muscle coverage using both the pectralis major and serratus anterior muscle would decrease the risk of infection, this technique may prevent smooth expansion, especially in the lower pole of the breast, thereby resulting in a high-riding device placement [10]. In the case of the breast with ptosis, the pectoralis major muscle alone is insufficient to cover the lower pole of the implant. Thus, the implant comes into direct contact with the skin, and that potentially causes ischemia of the skin. Breast surgeons in the USA are trying to overcome this anatomical limit by using Alloderm® [11, 12]. Absorbable materials should be resorbed at 3 to 4 weeks. If this happens, the implant will always come into direct contact with the skin. Using mesh sling or anchoring strings cannot improve the blood flow in the flap. But it is the same with Alloderm®. Then why does a sling with Alloderm® prevent capsular contracture [8, 13]? Iwahira said that the muscle envelope of the implant at the inferolateral site is not indispensable if the skin flap in there is sufficiently thick [14]. She also advocated that applying the serratus anterior muscle for the implant envelope would cause not only insufficient projection by the shortening of the lower part, but postoperative pain, or implant displacement. It is important that the implant is covered by a solid capsule with good blood flow. It does not matter if the muscle is there or not. The results of our present study seem to support this.

For studies of prosthesis-based breast reconstruction, extended follow-up is mandatory, as many complications, especially capsular contracture, develop long after the initial operation. We will continue to follow up with the patients of this study from this perspective. Nonetheless, once esthetics are compromised during the primary surgery, it will not improve spontaneously thereafter. Since DTI should be performed only in one operation, there is no opportunity for revision. For this decade, we performed the 158 DTI reconstruction with using absorbable materials and have never suffered from capsular contracture from early perioperative period. While performing DTI reconstruction using absorbable mesh sling technique and absorbable strings anchoring technique, we have got satisfaction about the results, both cosmetically and safely.

4.2 Direct-to-implant or taking two steps reconstruction

In this work, we introduced a unique DTI breast reconstruction technique that we developed with reference to Tessler's procedure. As a matter of fact, only these techniques can be practiced in our country where Alloderm® cannot be used. Long-term outcomes are yet to be accessed, but from the viewpoint of perioperative complications, safety appears acceptable in clinical practice.

In June 2013, the Japanese Central Social Insurance Medical Council of the Ministry of Health, Labor and Welfare approved insurance coverage for implants (prosthesis) used in breast reconstruction surgery, and insurance coverage began on July 1. The Japanese Society of Breast Oncoplastic Surgery began to collect data [15] from 2013, and then, there were 1281 cases undergone the breast reconstruction. With the exception of 2019, when breast implant-associated anaplastic large cell lymphoma (BIA-ALCL) gained public attention, the number of prosthesis breast reconstruction surgeries has continued to augment every year.

As described in "introduction", prosthesis-based breast reconstructive surgeries covered by insurance are classified into DTI and two-stage reconstruction. In the social burden of hospital visits, duration of hospitalization, and the medical costs associated with surgery, DTI reconstruction is superior. However, not only in Japan but also in the rest of the world, breast reconstruction is performed in two-stage.

According to aggregate results enforced by the Japanese Society of Breast Oncoplastic Surgery, the latest statistics in 2021 show that 388 cases were reconstructed in DTI manner, while 3667 cases were reconstructed in two-stage. The difference between the DTI and two-stage is almost ten times, and it can be said that two-stage reconstruction is the standard surgical procedure in Japan, de facto.

Japanese public insurance covered both DTI and two-stage breast reconstruction. In addition, two-stage reconstruction is clearly inferior in terms of patient burden than DTI manner. Why does as many as 90% of the surgeon select two-stage manner and DTI manner only 10%?

There are two notable papers.

The first is a big data study of 941,191 breast reconstruction cases after total mastectomy in the United States published by Kamali et al. in 2016 [16]. Using the Nationwide Inpatient Sample Database in the United States, they analyzed almost all patients who underwent DTI and two-stage reconstructive surgery, and investigated the basis for the selection of the two surgical procedures investigated. In the United States, 13.6% patients underwent DTI and 86.4%, two-stage reconstruction. As a result, DTI reconstruction is more likely to be selected for in the case of bilateral breast surgery. This reason is a patient factor. However, the patients, being nonwhite, being on Medicare, and living in a relatively western region, underwent DTI manner more often significantly. These factors could not be understood as a patient factor but should be accepted as rather a social factor. Two-stage reconstruction is more likely to be selected for patients aged 60 or over, which is a patient factor. However, two-stage reconstruction is more likely to be selected for patients; black, Hispanic, the person live in urban, undergoing surgery at the facility of the educational institution such as a university hospital, and are on Medicaid. Kamali said that the rationale for deciding the surgical manner, which was found to be highly significant by statistical processing, was not any patients' physical or disease-related factors, but more social reasons such as race and household income.

University hospitals and large facilities in urban areas are the centers of dissemination of information that determines a trend of the times. In these facilities, young doctors receive training of two-stage reconstruction manner as a standard. The ratio of doctors accustomed to two-stage manner and those accustomed to the DTI manner is 9:1, therefore the ratio of the patients underwent two-stage reconstruction and those underwent DTI reconstruction come down to 9:1. Most surgeons simply follow and perform the familiar procedure because the trend of the surgical manner of reconstruction in the past was so. As my interpretation of Kamali's work, that is thought to be the real reason why two-stage manner continues to be mainstream up to now.

The second important paper was published by Dikmans et al. in Lancet Oncology in 2017 [17]. This study was a prospective, randomized, multicenter, Phase IV trial designed to conclude the superiority of DTI versus two-stage reconstruction. As a result, it was revealed that DTI reconstruction was associated with a three-fold risk of perioperative complications (Odds 3.81, 95% CI 2.67–5.43, $p < 0.001$) and a risk of implant removal. Was eight times higher (8.80, 8.24–9.40, $p < 0\ 001$). By this work, this dispute which is a better manner between DTI and two-stage seems to have settled. Compared to two-stage reconstruction, DTI reconstruction has more complications and a higher risk of failure. We should select two-stage manner even if the disadvantages such as hospitalization and cost related to surgery are considered.

However, after considering this chapter in detail, it is unreasonable to apply this conclusion to clinical practice. The first point is breast size undergoing the reconstruction. Indeed, women's breasts in Japan may be relatively small compared to those in the United States. The average size of implants used in our hospital for breast reconstruction was 233.4 (80–595) ml (out of 205 cases). On the other hand, the average implant size used in Dikmans study was 392.1 or 416.2 ml in each group, and then, these averages were almost double the size of ours. The larger and heavier size of implant should cause the greater weight-bearing stress, especially in the lower half of the breast where the pectoralis major muscle defect. This condition compromises flap blood flow and increases complications. DTI is not suitable for reconstructing large mammary glands. Randomizing surgical procedures without considering breast size becomes disadvantageous to DTI.

Being with an incomplete muscle capsule is disadvantageous of DTI manner. Dikmans study also included currently smokers in 20% of DTI group and 13% of two-stage group. A decrease in skin flap blood flow due to smoking habit should increase ischemic complications, especially in DTI cases. Smoking cessation should be strictly enforced before surgery. Smoking cessation failures suggest that the patient's cooperation was not obtained in postoperative wound management, which is very important in reconstructive surgery with implants. This is especially true if the ratio of the smoker is higher in the DTI reconstruction group.

In this chapter, implant removal in the DTI group reached 11% of the total, but the expander removal rate in Two-stage was only 3%. However, 11% result is too high. The tabulated results of the Japanese Society of Breast Oncoplastic Surgery in Japan showed that the rate of implant removal in DTI group is 4.1% and in Two-stage is 3.8%, respectively [15]. In our result, the rate of implant removal in DTI was 3/158 cases (1.9%). Compared to these data, the outcomes of DTI reconstruction in Dikmans study was unnaturally bad. Again, the following factors may have contributed that the ratio of doctors accustomed to two-stage manner are nine-folds high to that accustomed to DTI manner. However, if you do not take any factors (breast size, smoker, surgeon proficiency) into consideration and choose a procedure at random, there is no doubt that you should definitely choose two-stage.

In Japan, where Alloderm® is not practical, the technology for DTI reconstruction has not been developed and never been trained. However, Tessler's method, our anchoring method using absorbable strings, can be practiced. Compared to the Tessler method, our method succeeded in lowering the possibility of SSI while retrospectively and with fewer observations.

Regarding the superiority of DTI reconstruction and two-stage reconstruction, a conclusion may eventually be drawn from the accumulation of big data in Japan. However, as Dikmans indicated, we must carefully select suitable patients for DTI reconstruction, and otherwise, we must be prepared for serious and highly frequent complications. In the current situation, patient selection criteria for DTI have not yet been established. From the patient's point of view, the DTI manner is clearly attractive because at the time when breast cancer surgery is over, and when she waked up from general anesthesia, the breast has already been reconstructed. No conclusions can be drawn until a situation arises in which a randomized trial is conducted at a facility with operators who are sufficiently familiar with both DTI and two-stage reconstruction. Until then, we must not abandon the pursuit and training of DTI reconstruction techniques just because we are unfamiliar with them.

Author details

Naoki Watanabe[1*], Shoko Otsuka[2], Sena Hori[3], Haruyuki Takata[4] and Takeshi Yuasa[5]

1 Nishihara Breast Clinic, Himeji, Japan

2 Department of Breast Surgery, Japanese Red Cross Society Himeji Hospital, Himeji, Japan

3 Hori Sena Breast Clinic, Obstetrics and Gynecology & Breast Clinic, Kobe, Japan

4 Department of Plastic Surgery, Japanese Red Cross Society Himeji Hospital, Himeji, Japan

5 Yuasa Breast Clinic, Kakogawa, Japan

*Address all correspondence to: nishihara.bs.clinic@lagoon.ocn.ne.jp

IntechOpen

© 2023 The Author(s). Licensee IntechOpen. This chapter is distributed under the terms of the Creative Commons Attribution License (http://creativecommons.org/licenses/by/3.0), which permits unrestricted use, distribution, and reproduction in any medium, provided the original work is properly cited.

References

[1] Hashimoto Y, Watanabe N, Yuasa T, Suzuki Y, Saisho H. Breast reconstruction with absorbable mesh sling: Dynamic infrared thermography of skin envelope. Gland Surgery. 2017;**6**(1):73-81. DOI: 10.21037/gs.2016.12.01

[2] Watanabe N. Clinical Practice of Direct-to-implant Breast Reconstruction for Breast Surgeon (only in Japanese): Gendaitosho Inc. 2017. 178 p. ISBN: 978-4-86299-028-0

[3] Tessler O, Reish RG, Maman DY, Smith BL, Austen WG Jr. Beyond biologics: Absorbable mesh as a low-cost, low-complication sling for implant-based breast reconstruction. Plastic and Reconstructive Surgery. 2014;**133**(2):90e-99e. DOI: 10.1097/01.prs.0000437253.55457.63

[4] Faulkner HR, Shikowitz-Behr L, McLeod M, Wright E, Hulsen J, Austen WG Jr. The use of absorbable mesh in implant-based breast reconstruction: A 7-year review. Plastic and Reconstructive Surgery. 2020;**146**(6):731e-736e. DOI: 10.1097/PRS.0000000000007384

[5] Institute NC. Common Terminology Criteria for Adverse Events (CTCAE). Japanese ed. U.S.A.: National Cancer Institute; 2017 [updated July 30, 2018 by JCOG. Version5.0:]. Available from: http://www.jcog.jp/doctor/tool/CTCAEv5.0J_20180915_miekeshi_v21_1.pdf (Original site) https://ctep.cancer.gov/protocolDevelopment/electronic_applications/ctc.htm#ctc_50

[6] Kanda Y. Investigation of the freely available easy-to-use software 'EZR' for medical statistics. Bone Marrow Transplantation. 2013;**48**(3):452-458. DOI: 10.1038/bmt.2012.244

[7] Colwell AS, Damjanovic B, Zahedi B, Medford-Davis L, Hertl C, Austen WG Jr. Retrospective review of 331 consecutive immediate single-stage implant reconstructions with acellular dermal matrix: Indications, complications, trends, and costs. Plastic and Reconstructive Surgery. 2011;**128**(6):1170-1178. DOI: 10.1097/PRS.0b013e318230c2f6

[8] Salzberg CA, Ashikari AY, Koch RM, Chabner-Thompson E. An 8-year experience of direct-to-implant immediate breast reconstruction using human acellular dermal matrix (AlloDerm). Plastic and Reconstructive Surgery. 2011;**127**(2):514-524. DOI: 10.1097/PRS.0b013e318200a961

[9] Cunningham B, McCue J. Safety and effectiveness of Mentor's MemoryGel implants at 6 years. Aesthetic Plastic Surgery. 2009;**33**(3):440-444. DOI: 10.1007/s00266-009-9364-6

[10] Namnoum JD. Expander/implant reconstruction with AlloDerm: Recent experience. Plastic and Reconstructive Surgery. 2009;**124**(2):387-394. DOI: 10.1097/PRS.0b013e3181aee95b

[11] Liu AS, Kao HK, Reish RG, Hergrueter CA, May JW Jr, Guo L. Postoperative complications in prosthesis-based breast reconstruction using acellular dermal matrix. Plastic and Reconstructive Surgery. 2011;**127**(5):1755-1762. DOI: 10.1097/PRS.0b013e31820cf233

[12] Komorowska-Timek E, Oberg KC, Timek TA, Gridley DS, Miles DAG. The effect of AlloDerm envelopes on periprosthetic capsule formation with and without radiation. Plastic and Reconstructive Surgery.

2009;**123**(3):807-816. DOI: 10.1097/PRS.0b013e318199eef3

[13] Gdalevitch P, Ho A, Genoway K, Alvrtsyan H, Bovill E, Lennox P, et al. Direct-to-implant single-stage immediate breast reconstruction with acellular dermal matrix: Predictors of failure. Plastic and Reconstructive Surgery. 2014;**133**(6):738e-747e. DOI: 10.1097/PRS.0000000000000171

[14] Iwahira Y, editor. Breast Reconstruction with Expander/Implant. 1st ed. Tokyo, Japan: Kanehara shuppan; 2014

[15] Surgery JSoBO. Annual Report on Usage Survey of Breast Implant and Tissue Expander in Japan, and its Complication (Japanese Only) Tokyo, JAPAN: Japanese Society of Breast Oncoplastic Surgery; 2013 [Available from: http://jopbs.umin.jp/medical/guideline/docs/gappeisho2013.pdf.

[16] Kamali P, Koolen PGL, Ibrahim AMS, Paul MA, Dikmans RE, Schermerhorn ML, et al. Analyzing regional differences over a 15-year trend of one-stage versus two-stage breast reconstruction in 941,191 Postmastectomy patients. Plastic and Reconstructive Surgery. 2016;**138**(1):1e-14e. DOI: 10.1097/PRS.0000000000002267

[17] Dikmans RE, Negenborn VL, Bouman MB, Winters HA, Twisk JW, Ruhe PQ, et al. Two-stage implant-based breast reconstruction compared with immediate one-stage implant-based breast reconstruction augmented with an acellular dermal matrix: An open-label, phase 4, multicentre, randomised, controlled trial. The Lancet Oncology. 2017;**18**(2):251-258. DOI: 10.1016/S1470-2045(16)30668-4

Chapter 5

Meshes in Implant-Based Breast Reconstruction: The Science and Technology

Emily Louise Hopwood, Annabelle Xiao Yan Tan and Fiona Jane Tsang-Wright

Abstract

Breast reconstruction is a common choice post mastectomy or breast-conserving surgery for breast cancer. Reconstructive options currently include implant-based and autologous reconstruction, with adjunctive use of surgical meshes. Acellular dermal matrices (ADMs) of both human and animal origin, and synthetic meshes are well-established for use in implant reconstruction. With ADMs, there is reduced risk of capsular contracture, providing a strong scaffold for prosthetic-based immediate reconstruction. Reduced seroma formation and infection has been demonstrated with synthetic mesh, thus both techniques proving advantageous. Use of mesh in implant-based reconstruction is a quickly evolving field, with hybrid meshes, 3D printed meshes and antibiotic-loaded meshes being investigated within the current literature. Whilst these surgical techniques are relatively new, they provide a new approach to many of the ethical issues currently surrounding use of surgical mesh.

Keywords: breast cancer, breast reconstruction, implant reconstruction, acellular dermal matrices, synthetic mesh, meshed enhanced hammock

1. Introduction

Breast cancer is one of the most prevalent malignancies in the UK, with 55,000 women and 370 men diagnosed every year in the UK alone [1]. Lifetime risk for women in the UK is currently one in seven, with breast cancer accounting for approximately 50% of all cancer diagnoses in women between the ages of 45–54 years old [2].

Breast cancer involves the breast tissue and may be invasive or non-invasive, with ductal carcinoma in situ (DCIS) being the most common subtype [3]. Current management for breast cancer in the UK may involve breast-conserving surgery or mastectomy, dependent on subtype and whether invasive disease is present [4]. Mastectomy is removal of the breast tissue and may be superseded by adjunctive radiotherapy, which has been demonstrated across the literature to reduce recurrence and mortality in women with lymph node involvement [5]. Following mastectomy, women may opt for delayed or immediate reconstruction, with the current trend in

IntechOpen

England towards immediate reconstruction, of which implant-based reconstruction accounts for 53% of cases in the UK [6]. Autologous reconstruction is another method, which may use the extended latissimus dorsi flap and provides good reconstruction for small to medium sized breasts [7]. Alternatively, the deep inferior epigastric perforator flap (DIEP) is another surgical technique deployed in breast reconstruction since 1994 [8] with added advantages of reduced ventral hernias and muscle weaknesses, previously seen with the free transverse rectus abdominus myocutaneous (TRAM) flap. In the TRAM flap, the TRAM muscle is removed from the abdomen and used to create the breast shape, whereas the DIEP flap creates the breast shape from tissue from the abdomen, sparing the abdominal muscle. The perforators of the deep inferior epigastric artery and vein are taken with the tissue and connected to the internal mammary artery and vein in the breast, advantageous due to increased sensory return of the breast compared to device-based reconstruction [9].

In early implant-based reconstruction, the implant was placed subcutaneously under the skin flaps and then the trend moved towards placing the implant in a pocket underneath the pectoralis major muscle [10]. However, there has been a change back to subcutaneous prepectoral implant insertions with the more widespread use of ADMs. There were initially increased complications pre-operatively [11]. Typically, tissue expanders are used first to expand the pocket under the pectoralis major muscle through a subcutaneous fluid injection, as this pocket is usually not large enough initially to house an implant [10]. Once the pocket has enlarged, the tissue expander is replaced in a further operation by a fixed volume implant. Newer combined expander implants can be used which is performed as one operation, reducing the number of operations required, and have good outcomes similar to other reconstructive methods [12] with low complication rates [13]. With an ADM more surgeons use a direct to implant approach, negating the use of a temporary expander in the prepectoral plane [14, 15].

Use of mesh as an adjunct in breast reconstructive surgery has been shown to have many advantages, providing a scaffold for host revascularisation and repopulation of cells, extending the pectoralis major muscle and space for the implant, thus forming a natural inframammary fold at the base of the implants [16]. Mesh reduces amount of tissue dissection required during surgery as well as the incidence of capsular contracture [17]. Despite this, they are also known to increase risk of seroma formation, skin necrosis, infection, and come at a high financial cost [18]. In a bid to reduce costs, use of absorbable vicryl mesh, alongside acellular dermal matrix (ADM), has been reported as safe and may provide a method to reduce material costs, without loss to the patient in terms of outcomes [19, 20].

2. History and development

Mesh, also referred to as 'matrices' is widely used across surgery in many different disciplines, including in abdominal and perineal wall closures, hernia repairs, colposuspension and rectoplexies. Prosthetic material was first suggested as a method to repair hernia defects in 1890 by Billroth [21] with original materials including silver metal braided as a weave, which led to problems surrounding toxicity due to silver sulphate formation on their surface [22].

Non-metallic materials were first considered for surgical use to repair defects by Koontz and Kimberly in 1959 [23]. However, the authors agreed that non-metallic materials may better fit the contours needing repair, thus should be considered in some circumstances [23]. Non-metallic materials including Dacron, Nylon and Teflon prove troublesome with infection, loss of tensile strength and rigidity [24], however tantalum gauze, a metallic material which used to be widely used in hernia repairs, escapes this. Marlex mesh was developed later, which had large pores thus incorporated well into tissue, with increased fibroblast activity and scaffold strength [25]. First generation meshes were introduced in 1998 and are based upon polypropene systems with large pores and small surface areas and are categorised into microporous, macroporous, and macroporous meshes with multifilament or microporous components [26].

Second generation meshes have increased tensile strength compared to their first generation counterparts [26]. They are composed of polypropylene (PP), polyester (PL) or expanded polytetrafluoroethylene (e-PTFE) combined with other materials such as titanium, omega 3, polyvinylidene fluoride (PVDF) and poliglecaprone 25 (PGC-25), and reduce formation of adhesions as the visceral and non-visceral sides of the mesh are specific to its function. The visceral side prevents adhesion through its microporous surface whilst the non-visceral side enables growth of parietal tissue through its macropores. Second generation meshes can be either absorbable or permanent.

The most recent development of surgical mesh encompasses those made from biological donor sources such as human dermis, bovine or porcine and greatly improve on the issues with second generation meshes, such as adhesion formation [26]. Human ADM was the first biological mesh produced and grafted well with tissues, with reduced rates of infection [27]. However, there are some issues with homografts, including increased risk of eventration, whereby a hernia forms at the same time as scars post surgery, with amount of stretch in the material also increasing over time [27]. Recurrence of hernias and fluid collections are also commonly seen after ADM use in abdominal wall reconstruction [28]. It has been thought in the literature that biological meshes reduce risk of capsular contracture when used in breast surgery, however have been associated with increased incidence of breast implant losses [29].

Matrices were first reported in the literature as being used in aesthetic breast revisions in 2003 to reduce rippling commonly seen with implant use [30], and in 2005 for breast reconstructions to reduce requirement for tissue expansion [31]. Following concerns raised by silicone-gel filled implants manufactured by PIP in 2010 [32], the safety of silicone-gel filled implants has been heavily investigated throughout the literature and they have been deemed as safe [33] and at present are the most common form of implant used in the UK for aesthetic breast augmentation [34] and breast reconstruction [35]. Matrices can be differentiated into biological ADMs and meshes [17]. ADMs are usually human, bovine or porcine derived and are soft tissue grafts containing only extracellular matrix after original cells are removed. They have been used in breast surgery since 2001, originally used for soft tissue coverage and as a structural scaffold for prosthetic-based immediate reconstruction [36] and utilise the prepectoral technique, described above (**Figure 1**) [37]. The patient's own cells will then revascularize the matrix, creating an additional tissue layer [17]. Contrastingly, there are synthetic meshes, which have comparable aesthetic outcomes to ADMs and are lower in cost [16]. Synthetic mesh has been used in breast reconstruction since 2005 with non-absorbable Mersilene mesh being the first [38]. Synthetic mesh is usually available as a sheet of plastic-like material with different

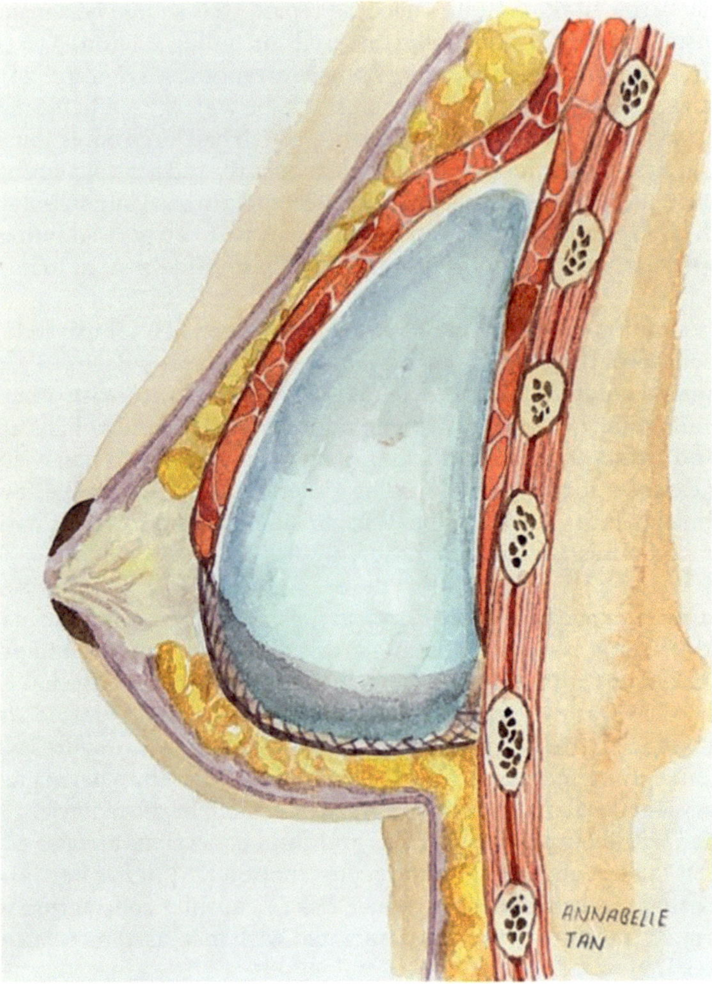

Figure 1.
Hand drawn image depicting subpectoral implant-based reconstruction [37].

sized pores dependent on mesh type, which affects how well the mesh is integrated into the breast tissue [39].

Within the prepectoral approach, ADMs can be used to recreate breasts when either a youthful appearance or ptotic breasts are desired, in a one-stage direct to fixed implant breast reconstruction [14]. The 'tent' technique, where the ADM is sutured to the pectoralis fascia can be utilised to create non-ptotic breasts; the 'enhanced hammock' technique allows for ptotic breast creation to recreate a similar breast where the alternate is already ptotic (**Figure 2**) [40], proving ADMs to be hugely versatile with regards to the final aesthetic appearance. The inferior free ADM edge is sutured a third up the implant edge on the pectoralis fascia, forming the 'hammock' [14]. Both of these techniques further promote a person-centred approach to implant-based reconstruction, with promising aesthetic results for patients due to superior breast symmetry.

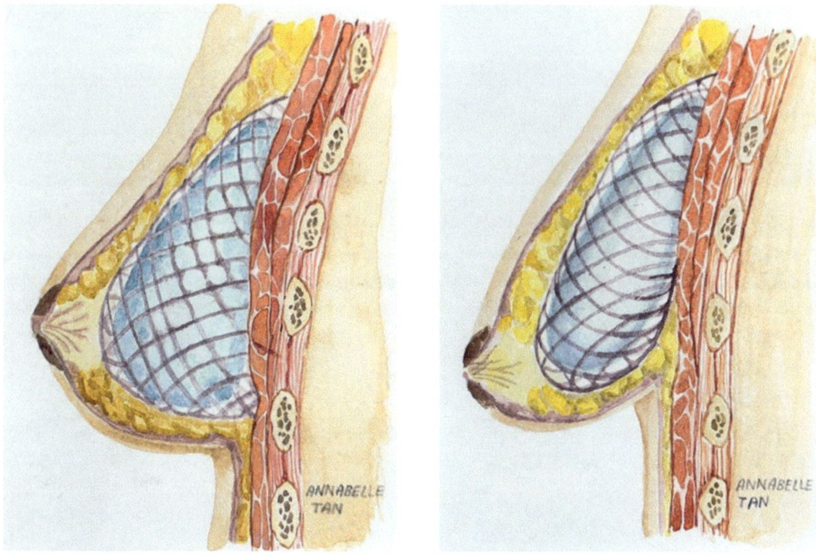

A B

Figure 2.
Hand drawn image showing prepectoral 'tent' (A) and 'enhanced-hammock' techniques (B) [40].

3. Current types

3.1 ADMS

In the UK, single stage direct to implant using animal derived ADM products is the most common form of implant reconstruction [15]. ADMs may be human, bovine or porcine derived and are composed of original dermal collagen matrix, which functions as a scaffold for revascularisation by the host's tissues [41]. Common sources of tissue used in ADM products (**Figure 3**) [42] include skin, small intestinal submucosa, amniotic membrane and peritoneal membrane [42]. First used in burns patients in the 1990s, they are currently applied in plastic and burns reconstructive surgery, skin grafts, orthopaedic surgery and breast reconstruction [42]. Whilst costly initially, they have been shown to be a cost-effective surgical technique with lower cost at 2 years post surgery [43].

3.2 Synthetic

Synthetic meshes are also used in breast reconstruction and are produced from plastic-like material and may be absorbable, non-absorbable or a mixture of both. Generally, they are lower in cost to ADMs [20]. Some studies have reported reduced or no infection or seroma formation post surgery with synthetic mesh, with aesthetic outcomes and patient satisfaction comparable with both synthetic and biological mesh [16, 44]. Synthetic meshes have poor incorporation into host tissue, which is one drawback to this surgical technique; of all synthetic materials used in meshes, PL is reported as having better incorporation [16].

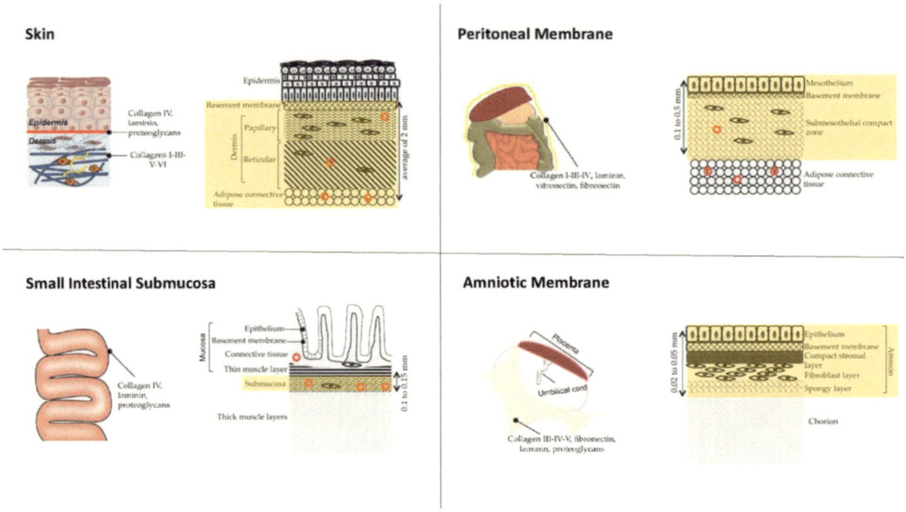

Figure 3.
Sources of ADM products [42].

3.3 Shapes

Meshes are available in different shapes, patches, plugs and sheets, all designed for various functions. Matrices may be knitted or woven; woven meshes have multiple parallel strands alternatively passed over and under another set of parallel strands, whilst knitted meshes are made using continuous loops of filaments [45]. Knitted meshes are the more traditional approach and are associated with increased post operative complications [46]. Patches and plugs are used in hernia repairs [26, 47], whilst flat sheet meshes are frequently used in implant-based breast reconstructions, notably sub-muscular and prepectoral reconstructions [48].

4. Indications

Popular indications for use of surgical mesh in breast surgeries are in implant-based total breast reconstructions post mastectomy, for patients with breast cancer or having risk reduction surgery, breast revision surgery, and surgery for congenital asymmetry or deformities. In the UK, biological and synthetic meshes have been used more frequently in ADM assisted procedures since 2013 [49]. Compared to traditional total submuscular techniques, mesh allows for better inframammary fold control and lower pole projection, with increased aesthetic results [50]. Synthetic meshes have been shown to be good substitutes for ADMs in aesthetic surgeries [51]. Lipomodelling is a more historical technique used to create symmetrical breasts in patients with congenital asymmetry [52]. Implants can be used in patients with amastia, uni-or bilateral absence of the breast and nipple-areola complex, Poland syndrome, where there is breast hypoplasia/aplasia and in tuberous breasts, where a fibrous ring blocks the radial development of the inferior mammary pole [53].

Risk reducing mastectomies may be chosen by women who are at higher genetic risk of developing breast cancer in their lifetime which may include those with the

BRCA1 or *BRCA2* genes or with a previous breast cancer diagnosis in the alternate breast [54] and is well reported as being the most effective way of reducing breast cancer risk in affected women [55]. *BRCA1* and *BRCA2* gene mutations increase a women's risk of breast cancer, with peak incidence at age 41–50 years in *BRCA1* carriers, and 51–60 years in *BRCA2* carriers [56]. For ovarian cancers, cumulative risk increases to 44% for *BRCA1* carriers and 17% for *BRCA2* carriers [56]. Risk reducing contralateral mastectomies have been illustrated as having a 48–63% survival advantage in patients with known *BRCA1* or *BRCA2* mutations [57, 58]. Implants may be placed prepectorally in these patients, and researchers argue that immediate reconstruction may be preferable to maintain self-esteem and aesthetic outcomes [55].

5. Complications

Common complications seen with surgical mesh use in breast reconstruction include infection, adhesion formation, capsular contracture and skin flap necrosis. Post operative adhesions can form after any type of surgery and carry increased risk of mortality and morbidity [59]. They increase operating time, as dissection can prove challenging, whilst can lead to patients requiring further surgeries to resolve [59]. There is currently poor understanding of the mechanism of adhesion formation with research suggesting the three main mechanisms include inhibition of extracellular and fibrinolytic degradation systems, an inflammatory response being induced by which cytokines and transforming growth factor-beta (TGF-beta) are produced, and tissue hypoxia, where vascular endothelial growth factor (VEGF) is expressed at increased levels [60]. Meticulous surgical technique is currently the gold standard prevention for adhesions, with liquid and solid anti-adhesive agents also able to be used, with limited evidence in laparoscopies [61].

Use of surgical mesh increases risk of site infection due to a prosthesis being introduced into the body, with risk post mastectomies being as high as 53% [62]. Notably, expander implants carried increased infection rates, compared to reconstructions using autologous tissues [63]. At present it is difficult to determine whether use of biological mesh in implant reconstruction leads to more complications [64], thus we must consider prevention of these complications. One trend to do this, is infection prophylaxis via antibiotics, alcohol-based skin preparation and pocket washout which feature in UK national guidance [15].

Capsular contracture commonly occurs post breast surgery due to an excessive fibrotic reaction to the foreign body known as the implant in the breast (**Figure 4**) [65], via an inflammatory response [66]. As a result, the collagen capsule that surrounds the implant contracts, distorting the breast tissue, and is categorised using the Baker classification system [67]. Class I describes a natural looking breast, II is a breast with minimal contracture, II, moderate contracture and IV, severe contracture [68] however recent literature reports poor reliability of this classification tool [69]. Capsular contracture can be caused by microbial biofilm formation [67], silicone or smooth implants, subglandular implant placement and prior radiotherapy to the breast [66]. At present, many techniques have been trialled to prevent and reduce risk of capsular contracture with breast implants post operatively, including use of biological and synthetic meshes adjunctively, anti-inflammatory and immune modulating drugs, anti-fibrotic drugs and antibiotics [65]. Physical modification of implants has been examined extensively and so research is now pointing towards pharmacological approaches in the hope that this will better reduce risk of capsular contracture.

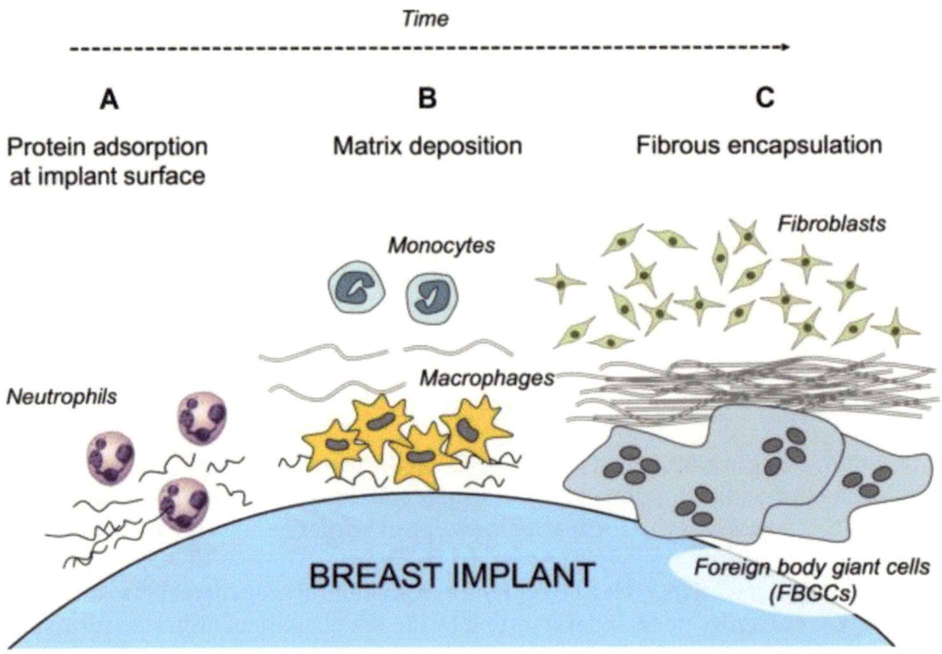

Figure 4.
Inflammatory response and foreign body reaction leading to capsular contracture [65].

Skin flap necrosis is another complication seen after implant reconstructions. Post mastectomy skin flap necrosis can lead to issues with wound management, infection of the implant and can look aesthetically displeasing [70]. The necrosis may be partial or full thickness and management can vary accordingly. Partial skin flap necrosis may require local wound care, whilst full thickness may need surgical debridement; it is known that adjunctive therapy such as chemotherapy or radiotherapy can be delayed if there is poor wound healing as a result of skin flap necrosis [70]. Risk factors for skin flap necrosis can include smoking, hypertension, increased breast volume [71–73]; modification of these pre-operatively may aid in reducing risk.

The long-term effects of the reconstructed breast, including breast symmetry, capsular contracture, infection rate, patient satisfaction, revisions and explantation rate are being evaluated in order to ascertain the long-term benefits and cost implications.

6. Future development

Surgical matrices are continually evolving, to suit the growing surgical requirements. Hybrid mesh, a mix of biological and synthetic materials are being explored further in the literature [27]. The combination is thought to combine the benefits of both materials, whilst reduce any complications they bring. Researchers believe that the biological part of the hybrid mesh, will protect the synthetic part from infection, and it is currently used in hernia repairs [27]. Hybrid meshes are seen as a cost-effective advancement in the field, with tensile strength of a synthetic mesh, but enabling for resorbable material to be used [74]. At time of writing, the literature presents us with limited evidence of this mesh in clinical practice, however no differences have been found in complication and recurrence rates between patients where synthetic and hybrid meshes were used [75]. Further research is required to fully evaluate the long-term effects in patients.

Biological meshes, being animal derived, bring into question some ethical issues, notably surrounding religious beliefs [76]. Animal derived products have been used in surgery for many years and we know that as a society composed of multiple religions and faiths, that animal products may spark important conversations. Porcine is the most common form of animal derived mesh, with bovine being the most accepted by religious groups in England [76]. This study highlighted the importance of clinicians having knowledge of the origins of their surgical meshes used, and how their patients' religious beliefs, if any, may translate across.

3D printed meshes may aid in alleviating this issue surrounding religious beliefs for biological mesh. Synthetic materials which are both biodegradable and biocompatible may be used in future 3D printed meshes, and this method would allow for personalised meshes to be quickly created, specific to each patient [77]. 3D printed meshes have already been considered in vaginal surgery [78] and hernia repairs [79], and are now being considered for use in breast reconstruction [80]. They offer an innovative new technology for reconstructive scaffolds with personalised breast shapes and sizes able to be created at a low cost, with the pore structure of the mesh providing access for fat injection at the implant site postoperatively [81]. One paper has shown 3D printed scaffolds as able to regenerate breast glandular tissue [82], an exciting advancement for their use in breast reconstructive surgery; as such, 3D printed scaffolds could be used to facilitate flapless nipple reconstruction when seeded with autologous adipose tissue and implanted subdermally at the site of reconstruction [83].

Drug loaded meshes are another recent advancement in the surgical field. Multiple studies have explored local antibiotic loading into mesh for infiltration into the surgical repair site [84–86]. Antibiotic delivery directly into the surgical site, reduces and prevents related infection [84], with antibiotics loaded onto the mesh surface [87]. Rifampicin, vancomycin and ciprofloxacin are some of the many antimicrobials which have been trialled [85, 86, 88]. To date, antibiotic loaded mesh has been explored for use in hernia [89] and vaginal repairs [78]. Looking ahead, this may enable for further development of loaded meshes in surgery; notably, stromal cells have been loaded onto a breast scaffold in breast reconstructive surgeries which led to a longer lasting graft, with increased vascularisation [90]. Whilst antibiotics can be loaded onto meshes, meshes can also gain antimicrobial properties via newer, alternative methods such as metallic particles [77], which have shown promise in recent studies [91–93].

7. Summary points

- Matrices are used in abdominal and perineal wall closures, hernia repairs, colposuspension and rectoplexies and breast reconstructive surgeries
- They may be biological (human, bovine or porcine derived) or synthetic, and are available in many shapes and sizes
- Complications are low

- 3D printing may pave the way for alternative forms of surgical mesh in the future
- Research supports the use of matrices in implant-based breast reconstruction, with early data supporting low complication rates and better cosmesis. New studies currently are underway to evaluate prepectoral implant-based reconstruction with or without a matrix.

Conflict of interest

The authors declare no conflict of interest.

Author details

Emily Louise Hopwood[1], Annabelle Xiao Yan Tan[2] and Fiona Jane Tsang-Wright[3*]

1 Buckinghamshire New University, High Wycombe, UK

2 University College London Medical School, London, UK

3 Buckinghamshire Healthcare NHS Trust, High Wycombe, UK

*Address all correspondence to: fiona.tsangwright@nhs.net

IntechOpen

© 2023 The Author(s). Licensee IntechOpen. This chapter is distributed under the terms of the Creative Commons Attribution License (http://creativecommons.org/licenses/by/3.0), which permits unrestricted use, distribution, and reproduction in any medium, provided the original work is properly cited.

References

[1] Breast Cancer Now. Facts and statistics 2021 [Internet]. 2021. Available from: https://breastcancernow.org/about-us/media/facts-statistics#:~:text=Around%2055%2C000%20women%20and%20370,are%20diagnosed%20with%20breast%20cancer [Accessed: 21 March 23]

[2] Office for National Statistics. Cancer registration statistics, England: 2017 [Internet]. 2019. Available from: https://www.ons.gov.uk/peoplepopulationandcommunity/healthandsocialcare/conditionsanddiseases/bulletins/cancerregistrationstatisticsengland/2017#links-to-related-statistics [Accessed: 21 March 23]

[3] Breast Cancer Now. Ductal carcinoma in situ (DCIS) [Internet]. 2023. Available from: https://breastcancernow.org/information-support/facing-breast-cancer/diagnosed-breast-cancer/primary-breast-cancer/ductal-carcinoma-in-situ-dcis [Accessed: 21 March 23]

[4] National Institute for Health and Care Excellence. Early and locally advanced breast cancer: Diagnosis and management [Internet]. 2018. Available from: https://www.nice.org.uk/guidance/ng101/resources/early-and-locally-advanced-breast-cancer-diagnosis-and-management-pdf-66141532913605 [Accessed: 21 March 23]

[5] McGale P, Correa C, Cutter D, Duane F, Ewertz M, Gray R, et al. Effect of radiotherapy after mastectomy and axillary surgery on 10-year recurrence and 20-year breast cancer mortality: Meta-analysis of individual patient data for 8135 women in 22 randomised trials. The Lancet. 2014;**383**(9935):2127-2135

[6] Mennie JC, Mohanna PN, O'Donoghue JM, Rainsbury R, Cromwell DA. National trends in immediate and delayed post-mastectomy reconstruction procedures in England: A seven-year population-based cohort study. European Journal of Surgical Oncology (EJSO). 2017;**43(1)**:52-61

[7] Chang DW, Youssef A, Cha S, Reece GP. Autologous breast reconstruction with the extended latissimus dorsi flap. Plastic and Reconstructive Surgery. 2002;**110**(3):751-759

[8] Allen RJ, Treece P. Deep inferior epigastric perforator flap for breast reconstruction. Annals of Plastic Surgery. 1994;**32**(1):32-38

[9] Huang H, Wang ML, Ellison A, Otterburn DM. Comparing autologous to device-based breast reconstruction: A pilot study of return in breast sensation. Annals of Plastic Surgery. 2022;**88**(3):184-189

[10] Potter S, MacKenzie M, Blazeby JM. Does the addition of mesh improve outcomes in implant based breast reconstruction after mastectomy for breast cancer? British Medical Journal (BMJ). 2018;**362**:1-14

[11] Yang JY, Kim CW, Lee JW, Kim SK, Lee SA, Hwang E. Considerations for patient selection: Prepectoral versus subpectoral implant-based breast reconstruction. Archives of Plastic Surgery. 2019;**46**(06):550-557

[12] Azzi AJ, Zammit D, Lessard L. Single-stage breast reconstruction using an all-in-one adjustable expander/implant. Plastic and Reconstructive Surgery Global Open. 2018;**6**(1):1609

[13] Goh SCJ, Thorne AL, Williams G, Laws SAM, Rainsbury RM. Breast reconstruction using permanent BeckerTM expander implants: An 18 year experience. The Breast. 2012;**21**(6):764-768

[14] Gui G, Tsang FJ. 'Meshed-enhanced hammock' or 'tent': A new patient centred pre-pectoral one-stage immediate breast reconstruction technique for varying ptosis. Annals of Plastic and Reconstructive Surgery. 2019;**3**(1):1-4

[15] Whisker L, Barber M, Egbeare D, Gandhi A, Gilmour A, Harvey J, et al. Biological and synthetic mesh assisted breast reconstruction procedures: Joint guidelines from the association of breast surgery and the British association of plastic, reconstructive and aesthetic surgeons. European Journal of Surgical Oncology. 2021;**47**(11):2807-2813

[16] Logan Ellis H, Asaolu O, Nebo V, Kasem A. Biological and synthetic mesh use in breast reconstructive surgery: A literature review. World Journal of Surgical Oncology. 2016;**14**(1):1-9

[17] Hallberg H, Rafnsdottir S, Selvaggi G, Strandell A, Samuelsson O, Stadig I, et al. Benefits and risks with acellular dermal matrix (ADM) and mesh support in immediate breast reconstruction: A systematic review and meta-analysis. Journal of Plastic Surgery and Hand Surgery. 2018;**52**(3):130-147

[18] Bank J, Phillips NA, Park JE, Song DH. Economic analysis and review of the literature on implant-based breast reconstruction with and without the use of the acellular dermal matrix. Aesthetic Plastic Surgery. 2013;**37**:1194-1201

[19] Karp NS, Salibian AA. Splitting the difference: Using synthetic and biologic mesh to decrease cost in prepectoral immediate implant breast reconstruction. Plastic and Reconstructive Surgery. 2021;**147**(3):580-584

[20] Tessler O, Reish RG, Maman DY, Smith BL, Austen WG Jr. Beyond biologics: Absorbable mesh as a low-cost, low-complication sling for implant-based breast reconstruction. Plastic and Reconstructive Surgery. 2014;**133**(2):90-99

[21] Billroth T. The Medical Sciences in the German Universities: A Study in the History of C. New York, NY, USA: Macmillan; 1924

[22] Idrees S, Jindal S, Gupta M, Sarangi R. Surgical meshes–the search continues. Current Medicine Research and Practice. 2018;**8**(5):177-182

[23] Koontz AR, Kimberly RC. Tantalum and marlex mesh (with a note on marlex thread): An experimental and clinical comparison—preliminary report. Annals of Surgery. 1960;**151**(5):796

[24] Usher FC, Fries JG, Ochsner JL, Tuttle LL. Marlex mesh, a new plastic mesh for replacing tissue defects. II. A new plastic mesh for replacing tissue defects. American Medical Association. Archives of Surgery. 1959;**78**:138-145

[25] Klinge U, Klosterhalfen B, Birkenhauer V, Junge K, Conze J, Schumpelick V. Impact of polymer pore size on the interface scar formation in a rat model. Journal of Surgical Research. 2002;**103**(2):208-214

[26] Baylón K, Rodríguez-Camarillo P, Elías-Zúñiga A, Díaz-Elizondo JA, Gilkerson R, Lozano K. Past, present and future of surgical meshes: A review. Membranes. 2017;7(3):47

[27] FitzGerald JF, Kumar AS. Biologic versus synthetic mesh reinforcement: What are the pros and cons? Clinics

in Colon and Rectal Surgery. 2014;**27**(04):140-148

[28] Patel KM, Bhanot P. Complications of acellular dermal matrices in abdominal wall reconstruction. Plastic and Reconstructive Surgery. 2012;**130**(5S-2):216-224

[29] Gschwantler-Kaulich D, Schrenk P, Bjelic-Radisic V, Unterrieder K, Leser C, Fink-Retter A, et al. Mesh versus acellular dermal matrix in immediate implant-based breast reconstruction–a prospective randomized trial. European Journal of Surgical Oncology (EJSO). 2016;**42**(5):665-671

[30] Duncan DI. Correction of implant rippling using allograft dermis. Aesthetic Surgery Journal. 2001;**21**(1):81-84

[31] Breuing KH, Warren SM. Immediate bilateral breast reconstruction with implants and inferolateral AlloDerm slings. Annals of Plastic Surgery. 2005;**55**(3):232-239

[32] Medicines and Healthcare products Regulatory Agency. Silicone gel filled breast implants- advice on clinical management of women with implants [Internet]. 2010. Available from: https://www.gov.uk/drug-device-alerts/medical-device-alert-silicone-gel-filled-breast-implants-advice-on-clinical-management-of-women-with-implants [Accessed: 9 April 23]

[33] Rohrich RJ, Kaplan J, Dayan E. Silicone implant illness: Science versus myth? Plastic and Reconstructive Surgery. 2019;**144**(1):98-109

[34] National Health Service. Breast enlargement (implants) [Internet]. 2023. Available from: https://www.nhs.uk/conditions/cosmetic-procedures/cosmetic-surgery/breast-enlargement/ [Accessed: 9 April 23]

[35] Breast Cancer Now. Breast Reconstruction [Internet]. 2018. Available from: https://breastcancernow.org/sites/default/files/publications/pdf/bcc7_reconstruction_2017_web.pdf/ [Accessed: 9 April 23]

[36] Salzberg CA. Nonexpansive immediate breast reconstruction using human acellular tissue matrix graft (AlloDerm). Annals of Plastic Surgery. 2006;**57**(1):1-5

[37] Tan AXY. Hand drawn image depicting subpectoral implant-based reconstruction. 2023

[38] Rietjens M, De Lorenzi F, Venturino M, Petit JY. The suspension technique to avoid the use of tissue expanders in breast reconstruction. Annals of Plastic Surgery. 2005;**54**(5):467-470

[39] Gómez-Modet S, Tejedor L. Synthetic mesh in immediate breast reconstruction. In: Gómez-Modet S, Tejedor L, Manchev L, Parikesit AA, editors. Breast Cancer and Breast Reconstruction. London: IntechOpen; 2020. pp. 141-159

[40] Tan AXY. Hand drawn image showing prepectoral 'tent' (A) and 'enhanced-hammock' techniques (B). 2023

[41] Sbitany H, Langstein HN. Acellular dermal matrix in primary breast reconstruction. Aesthetic Surgery Journal. 2011;**31**(7):30-37

[42] Petrie K, Cox CT, Becker BC, MacKay BJ. Clinical applications of acellular dermal matrices: A review. Scars, Burns & Healing. 2022;**8**:1-32

[43] Qureshi AA, Broderick K, Funk S, Reaven N, Tenenbaum MM, Myckatyn TM. Direct hospital cost of

outcome pathways in implant-based reconstruction with acellular dermal matrices. Plastic and Reconstructive Surgery Global Open. 2016;**4**(8):1-6

[44] Paganini A, Meyer S, Hallberg H, Hansson E. Are patients most satisfied with a synthetic or a biological mesh in dual-plane immediate breast reconstruction after 5 years? A randomized controlled trial comparing the two meshes in the same patient. Journal of Plastic, Reconstructive & Aesthetic Surgery. 2022;**75**(11):4133-4143

[45] Rastegarpour A, Cheung M, Vardhan M, Ibrahim MM, Butler CE, Levinson H. Surgical mesh for ventral incisional hernia repairs: Understanding mesh design. Plastic Surgery. 2016;**24**(1):41-50

[46] Kalaba S, Gerhard E, Winder JS, Pauli EM, Haluck RS, Yang J. Design strategies and applications of biomaterials and devices for hernia repair. Bioactive Materials. 2016;**1**(1):2-17

[47] Wu J, Wang Y, Yu J, Chen Y, Pang Y, Diao X, et al. Identification of implanted mesh after incisional hernia repair using an automated breast volume scanner. Journal of Ultrasound in Medicine. 2015;**34**(6):1071-1081

[48] Vidya R, Iqbal FM. A guide to prepectoral breast reconstruction: A new dimension to implant-based breast reconstruction. Clinical Breast Cancer. 2017;**17**(4):266-271

[49] Potter S, Conroy EJ, Cutress RI, Williamson PR, Whisker L, Thrush S, et al. Short-term safety outcomes of mastectomy and immediate implant-based breast reconstruction with and without mesh (iBRA): A multicentre, prospective cohort study. The Lancet Oncology. 2019;**20**(2):254-266

[50] Vardanian AJ, Clayton JL, Roostaeian J, Shirvanian V, Da Lio A, Lipa JE, et al. Comparison of implant-based immediate breast reconstruction with and without acellular dermal matrix. Plastic and Reconstructive Surgery. 2011;**128**(5):403-410

[51] Becker H, Lind JG. The use of synthetic mesh in reconstructive, revision, and cosmetic breast surgery. Aesthetic Plastic Surgery. 2013;**37**:914-921

[52] Derder M, Whitaker IS, Boudana D, Marchac A, Hivelin M, Mattar N, et al. The use of lipofilling to treat congenital hypoplastic breast anomalies: Preliminary experiences. Annals of Plastic Surgery. 2014;**73**(4):371-377

[53] Knackstedt R, Deross A, Moreira A. Congenital breast deformities: Anatomical basis and surgical approaches for optimal aesthetic outcomes. The Breast Journal. 2020;**26**(7):1302-1307

[54] Carbine NE, Lostumbo L, Wallace J, Ko H. Risk-reducing mastectomy for the prevention of primary breast cancer. Cochrane Database of Systematic Reviews. 2018;**4**:1-34

[55] Spindler N, Ebel F, Briest S, Wallochny S, Langer S. Quality of life after bilateral risk-reducing mastectomy and simultaneous reconstruction using pre-pectoral silicone implants. Patient Preference and Adherence. 2021:**15**:741-750

[56] Kuchenbaecker KB, Hopper JL, Barnes DR, Phillips KA, Mooij TM, Roos-Blom MJ, et al. Risks of breast, ovarian, and contralateral breast cancer for BRCA1 and BRCA2 mutation carriers. Journal of the American Medical Association (JAMA). 2017;**317**(23):2402-2416

[57] Evans DGR, Ingham SL, Baildam A, Ross GL, Lalloo F, Buchan I, et al. Contralateral mastectomy improves survival in women with BRCA1/2-associated breast cancer. Breast Cancer Research and Treatment. 2013;**2013**(140):135-142

[58] Metcalfe K, Gershman S, Ghadirian P, Lynch HT, Snyder C, Tung N, et al. Contralateral mastectomy and survival after breast cancer in carriers of BRCA1 and BRCA2 mutations: Retrospective analysis. British Medical Journal (BMJ). 2014;**348**:1-11

[59] Fatehi Hassanabad A, Zarzycki AN, Jeon K, Dundas JA, Vasanthan V, Deniset JF, et al. Prevention of post-operative adhesions: A comprehensive review of present and emerging strategies. Biomolecules. 2021;**11**(7):1027

[60] Coccolini F, Ansaloni L, Manfredi R, Campanati L, Poiasina E, Bertoli P, et al. Peritoneal adhesion index (PAI): Proposal of a score for the "ignored iceberg" of medicine and surgery. World Journal of Emergency Surgery. 2013;**8**(1):1-5

[61] Aref-Adib M, Phan T, Ades A. Preventing adhesions in laparoscopic surgery: The role of anti-adhesion agents. The Obstetrician & Gynaecologist. 2019;**21**(3):185-192

[62] Rubino C, Brongo S, Pagliara D, Cuomo R, Abbinante G, Campitiello N, et al. Infections in breast implants: A review with a focus on developing countries. The Journal of Infection in Developing Countries. 2014;**8**(09):1089-1095

[63] Pinsolle V, Grinfeder C, Mathoulin-Pelissier S, Faucher A. Complications analysis of 266 immediate breast reconstructions. Journal of Plastic, Reconstructive & Aesthetic Surgery. 2006;**59**(10):1017-1024

[64] Lardi AM, Ho-Asjoe M, Mohanna PN, Farhadi J. Immediate breast reconstruction with acellular dermal matrix: Factors affecting outcome. Journal of Plastic, Reconstructive & Aesthetic Surgery. 2014;**67**(8):1098-1105

[65] Guimier E, Carson L, David B, Lambert JM, Heery E, Malcolm RK. Pharmacological approaches for the prevention of breast implant capsular contracture. Journal of Surgical Research. 2022;**280**:129-150

[66] Headon H, Kasem A, Mokbel K. Capsular contracture after breast augmentation: An update for clinical practice. Archives of Plastic Surgery. 2015;**42**(5):532-543

[67] Ajdic D, Zoghbi Y, Gerth D, Panthaki ZJ, Thaller S. The relationship of bacterial biofilms and capsular contracture in breast implants. Aesthetic Surgery Journal. 2016;**36**(3):297-309

[68] Spear SL, Baker JL Jr. Classification of capsular contracture after prosthetic breast reconstruction. Plastic and Reconstructive Surgery. 1995;**96**(5):1119-1123

[69] de Bakker E, Rots M, Buncamper ME, Niessen FB, Smit JM, Winters HA, et al. The Baker classification for capsular contracture in breast implant surgery is unreliable as a diagnostic tool. Plastic and Reconstructive Surgery. 2020;**146**(5):956-962

[70] Robertson SA, Jeevaratnam JA, Agrawal A, Cutress RI. Mastectomy skin flap necrosis: Challenges and solutions. Breast Cancer: Targets and Therapy. 2017:**9**:141-152

[71] Downs RK, Hedges K. An alternative technique for immediate direct-to-implant breast reconstruction—a case series. Plastic and Reconstructive Surgery Global Open. 2016;**4**(7):1-8

[72] Ito H, Ueno T, Suga H, Shiraishi T, Isaka H, Imi K, et al. Risk factors for skin flap necrosis in breast cancer patients treated with mastectomy followed by immediate breast reconstruction. World Journal of Surgery. 2019;**43**:846-852

[73] Yalanis GC, Nag S, Georgek JR, Cooney CM, Manahan MA, Rosson GD, et al. Mastectomy weight and tissue expander volume predict necrosis and increased costs associated with breast reconstruction. Plastic and Reconstructive Surgery Global Open. 2015;**3**(7):1-9

[74] Rios-Diaz AJ, Hitchner M, Christopher AN, Broach R, Cunning JR, Fischer JP. Early clinical and patient-reported outcomes of a new hybrid mesh for incisional hernia repair. Journal of Surgical Research. 2021;**265**:49-59

[75] Kudsi OY, Kaoukabani G, Bou-Ayash N, Gokcal F. Comparison of hybrid versus synthetic mesh in robotic rives-stoppa ventral hernia repair. Journal of the Society of Laparoscopic & Robotic Surgeons (JSLS). 2022;**26**(4):1-11

[76] Koshy RM, Kane EG, Grocock C. A review of the use of biological mesh products in modern UK surgical practice: A religious and cultural perspective. The Annals of The Royal College of Surgeons of England. 2020;**102**(8):566-570

[77] Corduas F, Lamprou DA, Mancuso E. Next-generation surgical meshes for drug delivery and tissue engineering applications: Materials, design and emerging manufacturing technologies. Bio-Design and Manufacturing. 2021;**4**:278-310

[78] Domínguez-Robles J, Mancinelli C, Mancuso E, García-Romero I, Gilmore BF, Casettari L, et al. 3D printing of drug-loaded thermoplastic polyurethane meshes: A potential material for soft tissue reinforcement in vaginal surgery. Pharmaceutics. 2020;**12**(1):63

[79] Pérez-Köhler B, Benito-Martínez S, Gómez-Gil V, Rodríguez M, Pascual G, Bellón JM. New insights into the application of 3D-printing technology in hernia repair. Materials. 2021;**14**(22):7092

[80] Mu X, Zhang J, Jiang Y. 3D printing in breast reconstruction: From bench to bed. Frontiers in Surgery. 2021;**8**:641370

[81] Juliang Z, Qing Y, Meiling H, Mingkun Z, Huimin M, Lan H. Computer-assisted 3-dimensional printing technology for immediate breast reconstruction after breast-conserving surgery. Chinese Journal of Breast Disease. 2018;**12**:12-16

[82] Sokol ES, Miller DH, Breggia A, Spencer KC, Arendt LM, Gupta PB. Growth of human breast tissues from patient cells in 3D hydrogel scaffolds. Breast Cancer Research. 2016;**18**:1-13

[83] Khoo D, Ung O, Blomberger D, Hutmacher DW. Nipple reconstruction: A regenerative medicine approach using 3d-printed tissue scaffolds. Tissue Engineering Part B: Reviews. 2019;**25**(2):126-134

[84] Labay C, Canal JM, Modic M, Cvelbar U, Quiles M, Armengol M, et al. Antibiotic-loaded polypropylene surgical meshes with suitable biological behaviour by plasma functionalization and polymerization. Biomaterials. 2015;**71**:132-144

[85] Qamar N, Abbas N, Irfan M, Hussain A, Arshad MS, Latif S, et al.

Personalized 3D printed ciprofloxacin impregnated meshes for the management of hernia. Journal of Drug Delivery Science and Technology. 2019;**53**:101164

[86] Reinbold J, Hierlemann T, Urich L, Uhde AK, Müller I, Weindl T, et al. Biodegradable rifampicin-releasing coating of surgical meshes for the prevention of bacterial infections. Drug Design, Development and Therapy. 2017:2753-2762

[87] Pérez-Köhler B, Linardi F, Pascual G, Bellón JM, Eglin D, Guillaume O. Efficacy of antimicrobial agents delivered to hernia meshes using an adaptable thermo-responsive hyaluronic acid-based coating. Hernia. 2020;**24**:1201-1210

[88] Blatnik JA, Thatiparti TR, Krpata DM, Zuckerman ST, Rosen MJ, Von Recum HA. Infection prevention using affinity polymer-coated, synthetic meshes in a pig hernia model. Journal of Surgical Research. 2017;**2017**(219):5-10

[89] See CW, Kim T, Zhu D. Hernia mesh and hernia repair: A review. Engineered Regeneration. 2020;**1**:19-33

[90] Gentile P, Casella D, Palma E, Calabrese C. Engineered fat graft enhanced with adipose-derived stromal vascular fraction cells for regenerative medicine: Clinical, histological and instrumental evaluation in breast reconstruction. Journal of Clinical Medicine. 2019;**8**(4):504

[91] Chen P, Wu Z, Leung A, Chen X, Landao-Bassonga E, Gao J, et al. Fabrication of a silver nanoparticle-coated collagen membrane with anti-bacterial and anti-inflammatory activities for guided bone regeneration. Biomedical Materials. 2018;**13**(6):065014

[92] Dizaj SM, Lotfipour F, Barzegar-Jalali M, Zarrintan MH, Adibkia K. Antimicrobial activity of the metals and metal oxide nanoparticles. Materials Science and Engineering: C. 2014;**44**:278-284

[93] Muwaffak Z, Goyanes A, Clark V, Basit AW, Hilton ST, Gaisford S. Patient-specific 3D scanned and 3D printed antimicrobial polycaprolactone wound dressings. International Journal of Pharmaceutics. 2017;**527**(1-2):161-170

Chapter 6

Thoracoabdominal Flaps for Breast Reconstruction: Different Types and Classification

Ernesto A. Moretti

Abstract

The thoracoabdominal flaps allow the closure thoracic defects with a lower technical difficulty and morbidity compared to remote flaps. In mammary oncological reconstructive surgery, they were used primarily as fasciocutaneous flaps for patients with locally advanced breast cancer (T3 and T4 tumors) that require large skin resections and a fast and effective coverage of the thoracic defect. In recent years, they have resurged as a therapeutic option to solve postoperative complications due to ischemia and skin necrosis with exposure of tissue expanders or breast implants. The increase in the practice of risk-reducing mastectomies (RRM) has led to areas of small skin suffering or necrosis that require local flaps to solve the complication. It is in these indications, where these flaps have an optimal application. In the present study, the thoracoabdominal flaps are presented as a very useful reconstructive technique to cover skin defects in breast surgery complications. A classification is presented to clarify these fasciocutaneous flaps, as well as examples of their applications.

Keywords: thoracoabdominal flap, thoracoepigastric flap, breast reconstruction, surgery, complications

1. Introduction

The reconstruction of breast deformities secondary to procedures for oncological disease is still one of the main challenges of reconstructive plastic surgery. Immediate reconstruction with alloplastic materials is one of the most common alternatives for selected patients, who often prefer this type of surgery over reconstruction with more extensive and complex procedures that involve the use of autologous tissues [1]. However, the resection techniques and the adjuvant treatments for oncological surgery condition (particularly radiotherapy) frequently give a hostile and inadequate adaptation of the organism to implants and tissue expanders, producing in numerous cases the dehiscence of wounds, necrosis of the cutaneous tissues, and the exposure of the alloplastic material, risking the esthetic result of the surgery, and on unfortunate occasions, lead to the failure of the repair technique due to the need for explantation, producing a transient deformity that has a high emotional impact for the patient [2].

The thoracoabdominal flaps are one of the best known and most used flaps in breast reconstruction surgery, particularly in resolving complications.

This chapter details the thoracoabdominal flaps described in the literature, as well as clarifies their planning and rotation. A classification is presented to avoid confusion in the nomenclature.

2. History

The lateral pedicle thoracoabdominal flap or also called the lateral thoracodorsal flap is a rotation/transposition fasciocutaneous flap based on the posterior perforators of the intercostal vessels of the thoracodorsal vessels and was initially described by Hölmstrom and Lossing [3] in 1986. In their publication, the flap is combined with breast implants as an alternative to musculocutaneous flaps for breast reconstruction. The Hölmstrom technique is based on the description of the thoracoepigastric flap described by Cronin [4] and Bohmert [5], a technique that describes a similar flap but with a medial pedicle (based on the perforators of the superior epigastric artery).

The use of this lateral pedicle thoracoabdominal flap has had numerous publications in Scandinavian countries, where there are several publications [6–8]. In Latin America, although is less widespread, there are works published such as Pontes [9] from Brazil, Carriquiri [10] from Uruguay, and Fullana Sastre from Barcelona [11].

3. Anatomy of the toracoabdominal flaps

When considering the anatomy of the intercostal vessels, it is important to understand its origins. The intercostal vessels form an arcade between the aorta posteriorly and the internal mammary vessels anteriorly.

The arcade is divided into vertebral, costal, and muscular segments. In the lateral area of the thorax, the six, seven, and eight intercostal vessels give lateral anterior perforators (LICAP: lateral intercostal anterior perforator) that provide irrigation to the skin, subcutaneous tissues, and muscular fascias (**Figure 1**).

These perforators supply the anterior region of the thorax and abdomen below the lower outer quadrant (LOQ) of the mammary region. The intercostal vessels continue their internal course below the costal arches and deliver the second anterior perforators. This perforator is called AICAP (anterior intercostal perforator), which supplies the regions of the thorax and abdomen at the level of the lower inner quadrant (LIQ) of the mammary region (**Figure 2**).

These perforators of the intercostal vessels six, seven, and eight can be identified with echo Doppler, although they can constantly be marked in an imaginary vertical line from the submammary fold to the nipple-areola complex. Continuing along the route, the intercostal vessels join to the internal mammary or middle thoracic artery, closing the vascular circuit (**Figure 3**). This artery is a collateral vessel from the subclavian artery.

In this thoracoabdominal area below the lower internal quadrant of the breast, the middle thoracic artery delivers perforators at the level of the sixth costal arch and subsequently delivers perforators that cross the rectus abdominis muscle. In this area, the internal mammary artery changes name to the superior epigastric artery. These perforators supply the central part and lower inner quadrants of the thoracic region and upper hemiabdomen, making the MICAP perforators (Middle Intercostal Anterior Perforator) (**Figure 4**).

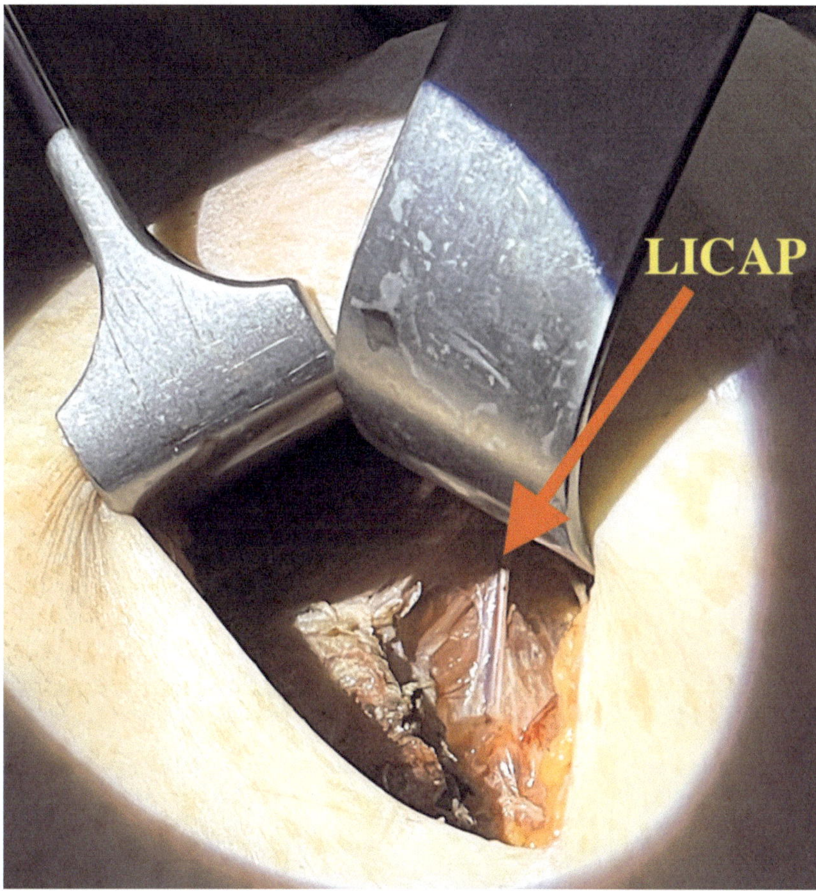

Figure 1.
Intraoperative image at the level of the submammary fold in its external area, where the lateral perforator of the intercostal vessels (LICAP) is marked (red arrow).

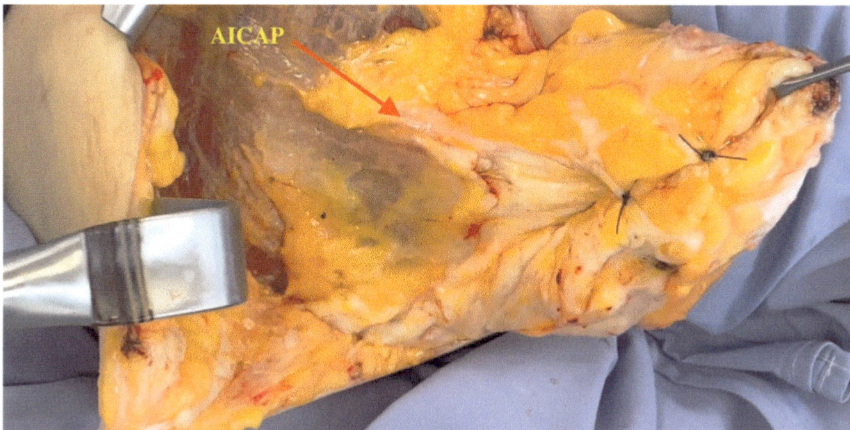

Figure 2.
Intraoperative image of breast reduction surgery, where the anterior perforating vessels of the fifth intercostal artery are observed (AICAP).

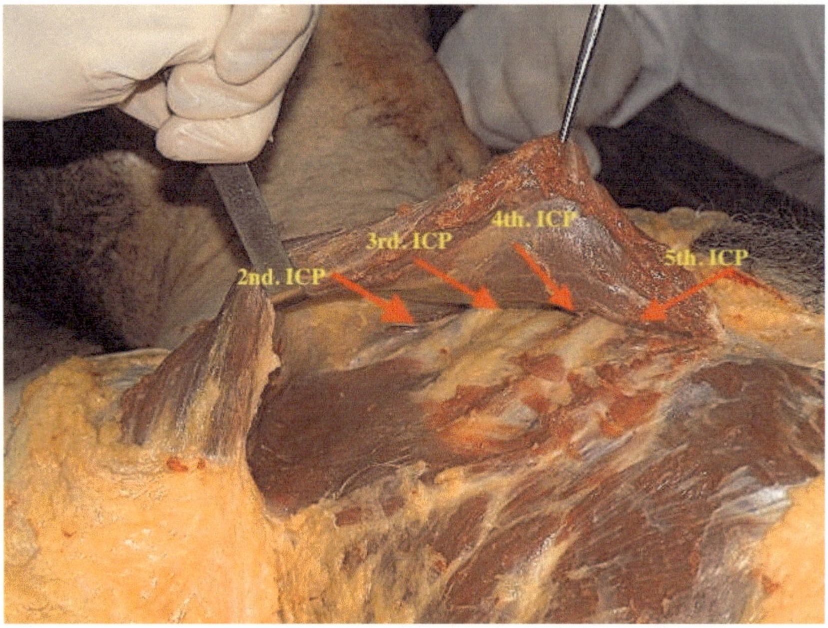

Figure 3.
Image obtained from fresh cadaveric dissection, where the second, third, fourth, and fifth intercostal arteries are observed in the direction of joining with the internal mammary artery. The red arrows show the perforators.

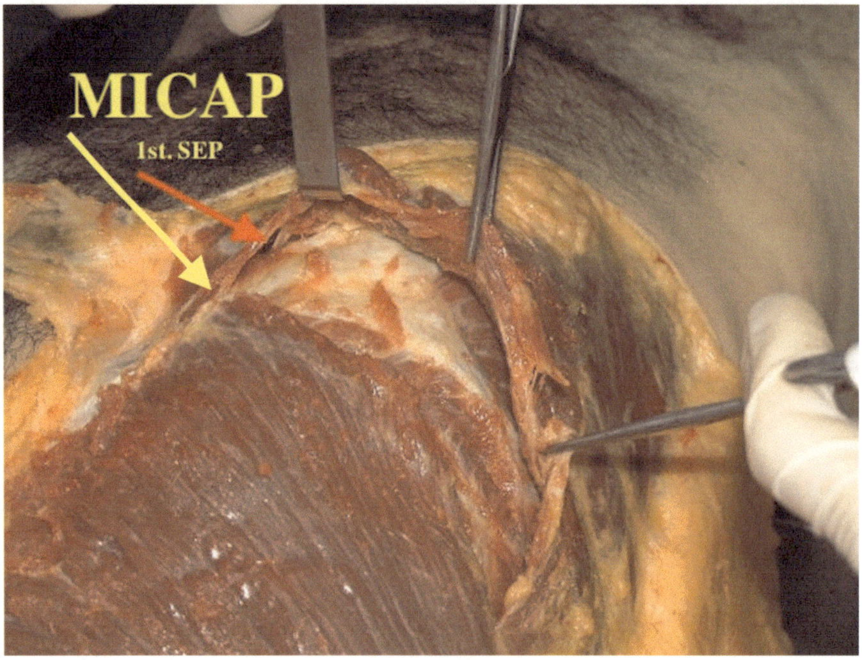

Figure 4.
Image where the first perforator of the superior epigastric artery is identified with a red arrow. This perforator comes from the internal mammary artery that changes its name when it crosses the diaphragm. The perforator of the sixth intercostal artery provides irrigation to the innermost sectors of the lower region of the thorax (MICAP) (yellow arrow). Anatomically, the perforators of the epigastric artery do not join the intercostal vessels.

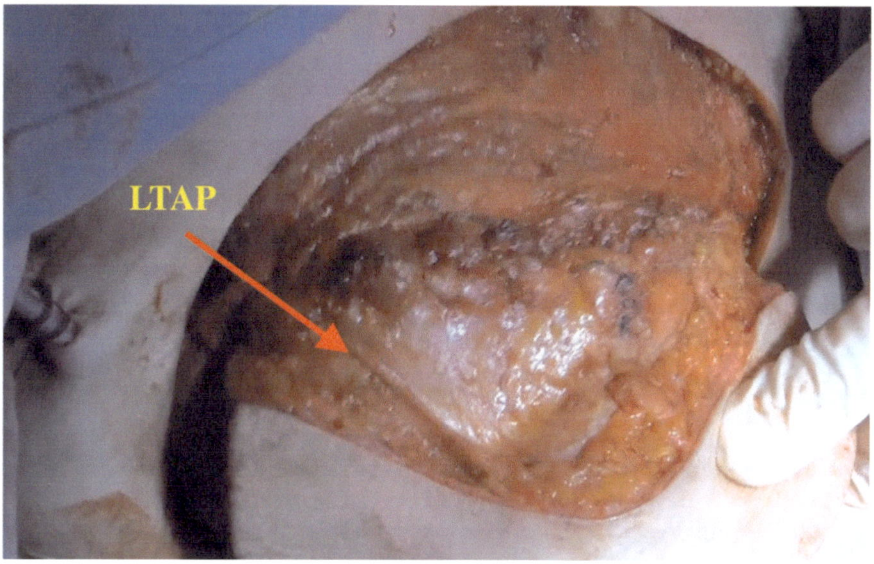

Figure 5.
Intraoperative image of breast reconstruction showing the lateral thoracic artery perforator, base of the fasciocutaneous flap LTAP.

It should also be mentioned that the lateral irrigation of the thorax and upper hemiabdomen receive irrigation from the lateral thoracic artery, which comes from the axillary artery, and delivers two to three perforators in its lower part, creating perforators called LTAP (lateral thoracic artery perforator) (**Figure 5**). These perforators supply the skin, subcutaneous tissue, and muscle fascia at the level of the midaxillary line in the region of the sixth, seventh, and eighth ribs.

In conclusion, the area of the chest wall beneath the inframammary fold and upper abdominal area can be divided into four regions. Medially, the medial intercostal artery perforator (MICAP) is present; centrally, the AICAP is present, and laterally, the LICAP and the LTAP are present.

4. Surgical variants

The following table classifies the fasciocutaneous flaps of the upper hemiabdomen and lower parts of the thorax. Different thoracoabdominal flaps and their surgical variants are listed.

5. Classification

5.1 Fasciocutaneous flaps of the upper hemiabdomen and lower part of the thorax

- TYPE I: Lateral Thoracoabdominal Flaps.

  - I A: Anterior rotation base (based on the TLAP).
  - I B: Posterior rotation base (based on the LICAP).
- TYPE II: Medial Thoracoabdominal Flap or Thoracoepigastric Flap (based on the MICAP and 1st SEP).
- TYPE III: Thoracoabdominal Island Flaps.
  - III A: Lateral rotation base (based on the LICAP).
  - III B: Medial rotation base (based on the MICAP).
- TYPE IV: Thoracoabdominal Dermofat Flaps.
  - IV A: Lateral rotation base (based on the LICAP).
  - IV B: Medial rotation base (based on the MICAP).

5.1.1 TYPE I: Lateral thoracoabdominal flaps

See **Figure 6**.

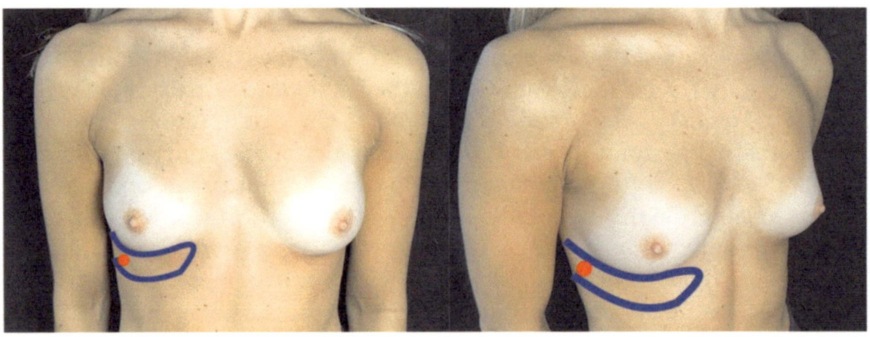

Figure 6.
TYPE I A: Anterior rotation base (based on the TLAP). Red dot indicates the location of perforating artery.

See **Figure 7**.

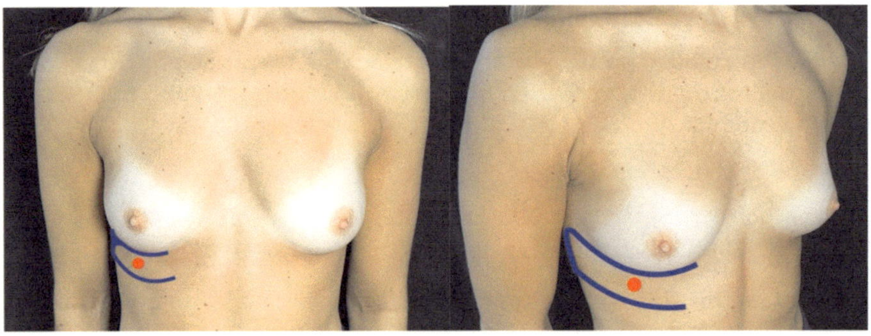

Figure 7.
TYPE I B: Posterior rotation base (based on the LICAP). Red dot indicates the location of perforating artery.

DOI: http://dx.doi.org/10.5772/intechopen.112912

5.1.2 TYPE II: Medial thoracoabdominal flap or thoracoepigastric flap

See **Figure 8**.

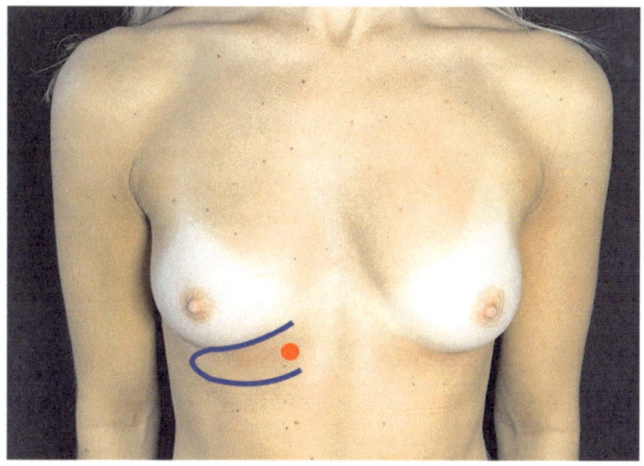

Figure 8.
TYPE II: Medial Thoracoabdominal Flap or Thoracoepigastric Flap (based on the MICAP and 1st SEP: red dot).

5.1.3 TYPE III: Thoracoabdominal Island flaps

See **Figure 9**.

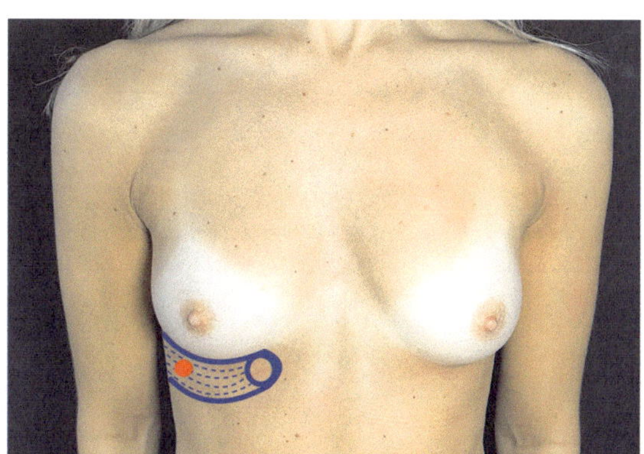

Figure 9.
TYPE III A: Lateral rotation base (based on the LICAP). Dotted lines indicate desepidermized area. Circular zone indicates the skin area to be transposed.

See **Figure 10**.

5.1.4 TYPE IV: Thoracoabdominal dermofat flaps

See **Figure 11**.
See **Figure 12**.

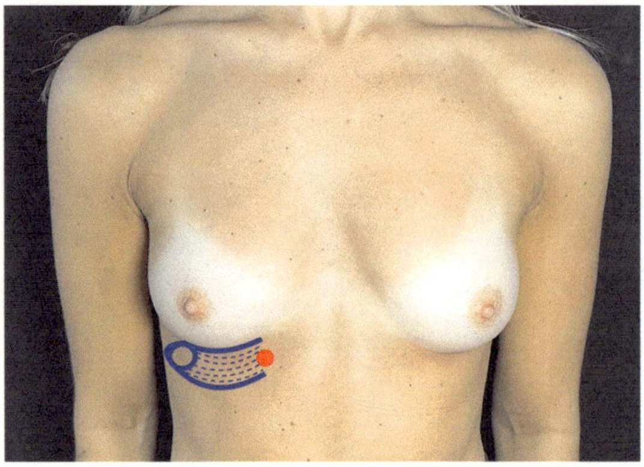

Figure 10.
TYPE III B: Medial rotation base (based on the MICAP). Dotted lines indicate desepidermized area. Circular zone indicates the skin area to be transposed.

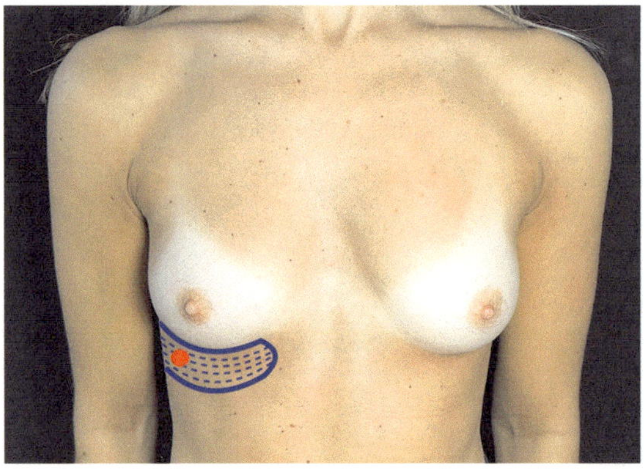

Figure 11.
TYPE IV A: Lateral rotation base (based on the LICAP). Dotted lines indicate desepidermized area.

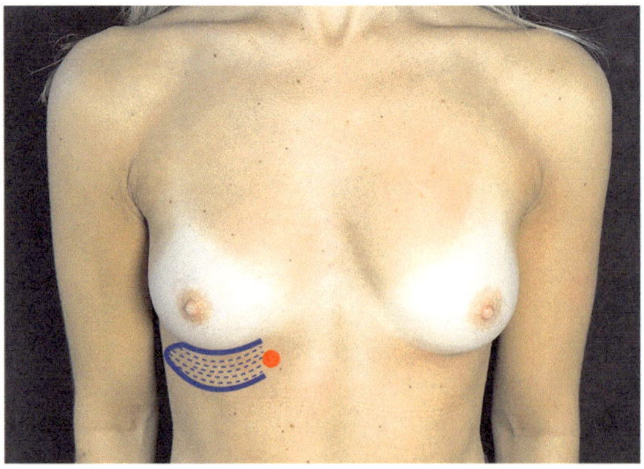

Figure 12.
TYPE IV B: Medial rotation base (based on the MICAP). Dotted lines indicate desepidermized area.

6. Fasciocutaneous flaps of the upper abdomen and lower part of the thorax

6.1 Clinical cases

6.1.1 TYPE I: Lateral thoracoabdominal flaps

The lateral thoracoabdominal flap or type I is a local flap that allows elevation and rotation of the skin, subcutaneous tissue, and fascia surface from the upper abdomen and lower part of the thorax. It is supplied by the perforators of the arteries tributaries of the lateral thoracic artery and the intercostal artery. It is a very versatile flap that allows to resolve local complications of the lower outer quadrant (LOQ) and/or medial region of the breast [12].

The initial description, as well as in most of the published works, uses the skin and subcutaneous tissues with the inner fascia (Superficial Fascia System — Fascia of Scarpa) provided from the lateral and posterior region of the thorax. In this way, the flap has an anterior base and rotates 90 degrees from back to front (CASE 1 and 2). The flap can also be used but with a posterior base. In this case, it provides tissues from the anterior region of the upper abdomen (CASE 3, 4, AND 5). It is, therefore, according to our classification, there are two variants of the lateral pedicle thoracoabdominal flap (**Figures 13–16**).

6.1.2 TYPE II: Medial thoracoabdominal flap or Thoracoepigastric flap

The thoracoabdominal axial flap to the medial pedicle or also frequently called "thoracoepigastric flap" is presented as an option for the local reconstruction of lesions in the lower inner quadrant (LIQ) of the breast. Its irrigation is given by the perforator of the middle thoracic artery, generally the sixth perforator, and perforators of the superior epigastric artery.

This flap exclusively has a base of rotation directed from the epigastrium, which is why it has no variants. It is a flap that allows the use of tissues from the upper hemiabdomen and contributes tissues to defects in the middle of the breast, especially to central areas and lower internal quadrants.

See **Figure 17**.

See **Figure 18**.

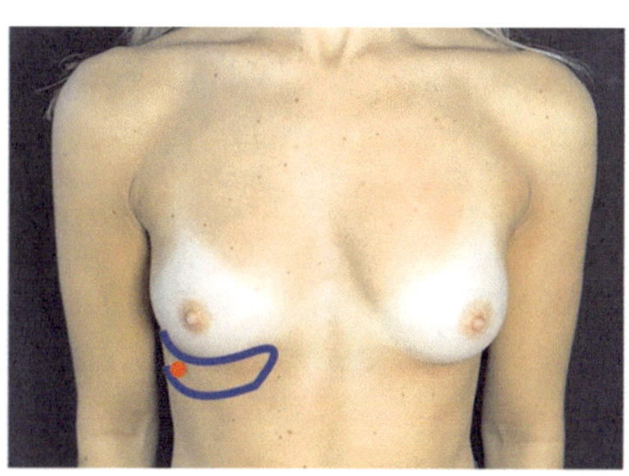

Figure 13.
TYPE I A: I A: Anterior rotation base (based on the TLAP).

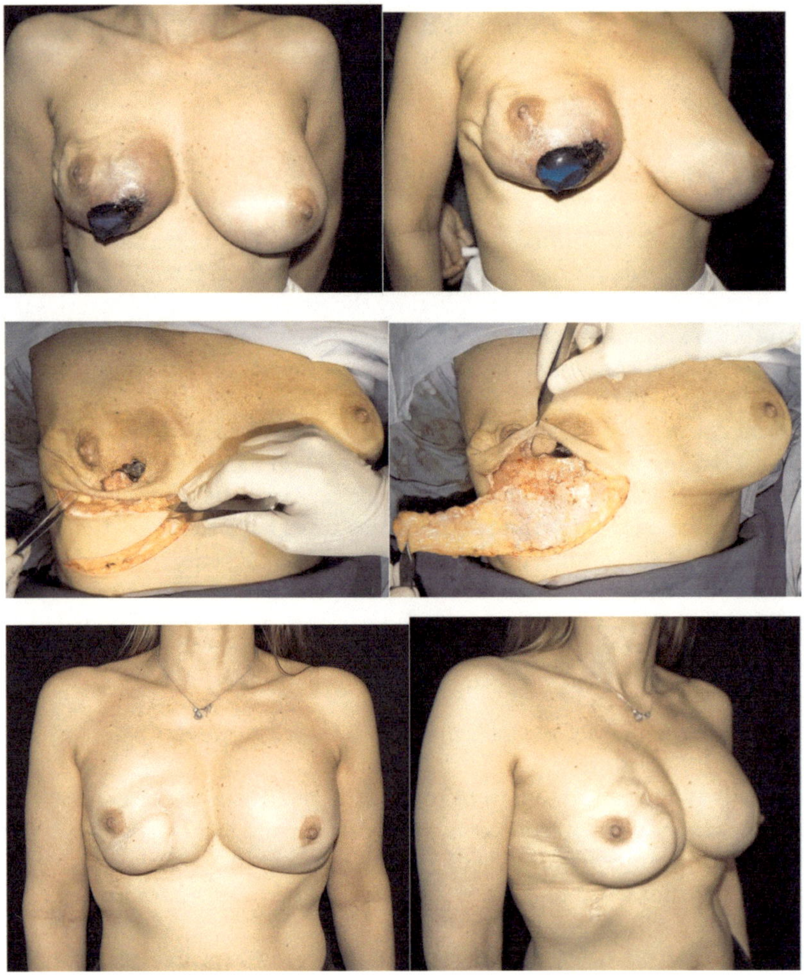

Figure 14.
36-year-old patient with right breast reconstruction in another institution. The patient was hospitalized in our hospital and immediately removed the expander. The TYPE I A flap was designed and applied in the area of the surgical defect. Three months later, an anatomically shaped implant was placed, and risk-reducing mastectomy (RRM) was performed in the left breast. Postoperative control images 1 year after the procedure.

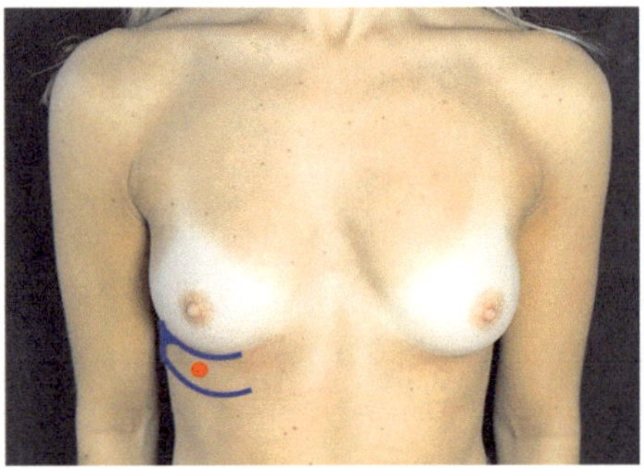

Figure 15.
TYPE I B: Posterior rotation base (based on the LICAP).

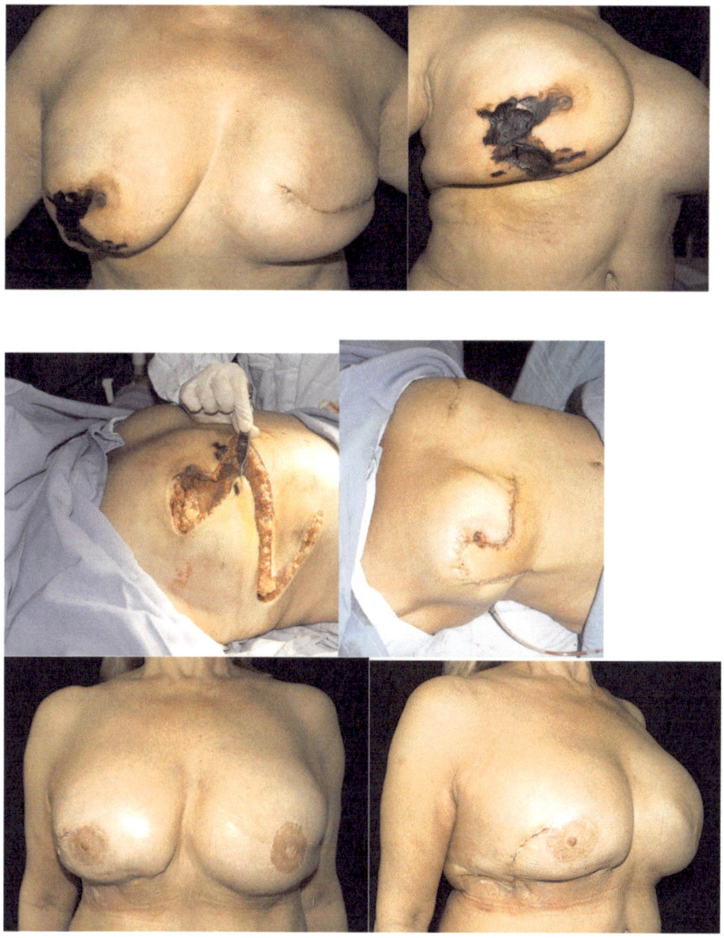

Figure 16.
66-year-old patient with left mastectomy and risk-reducing mastectomy were performed on the right breast. A well-defined area of skin necrosis in the right breast was observed after 10 days. No signs of infection. A TYPE IB thoracoabdominal flap was planned, preserving the implant placed in the first surgical procedure. Images were taken at 6 months with reconstruction of bilateral nipple-areola complexes and solution of the skin defect.

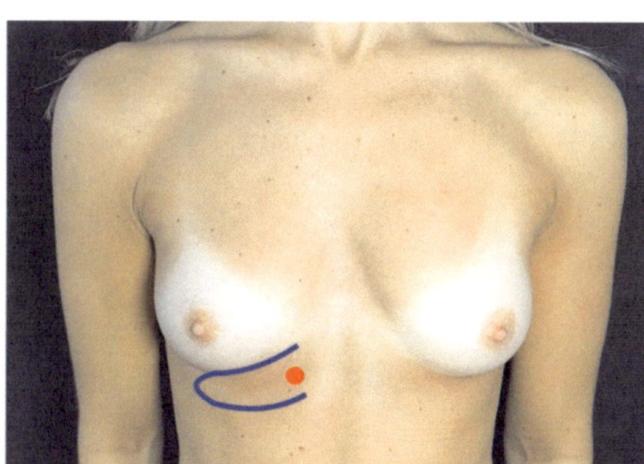

Figure 17.
TYPE II: Medial Thoracoabdominal flap or Thoracoepigastric flap.

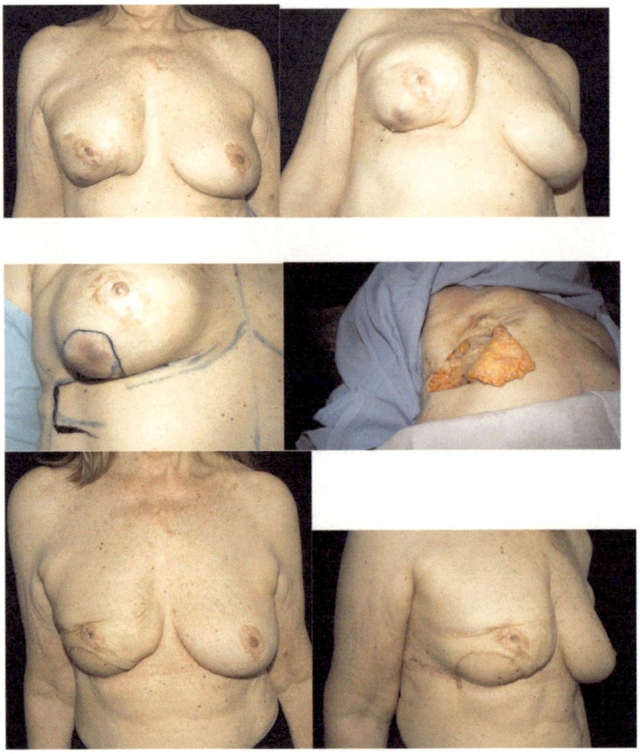

Figure 18.
68-year-old patient with 10 years postoperative right mastectomy for breast carcinoma and risk-reducing mastectomy of the left breast. She presented capsulitis with an inferior infection process and a tendency to decubitus of the implant placed. It was decided to remove the implant, toilette the area, plan a TYPE II thoracoepigastric flap, and place a new breast implant. Images obtained at 3 months with resolution of the problem.

6.1.3 TYPE III: Thoracoabdominal Island flaps

The thoracoabdominal island flap is described by Rose and Svensson [13] for small defects circumscribed to the inferior-external quadrant (Variant III A) and the inferior-internal quadrant (Variant III B). The length-to-width ratio of the flap should not be greater than 2:1 because it is an axial flap. The defect caused by the cutaneous island must be covered by an abdominal flap detaching to the subdermal plane.

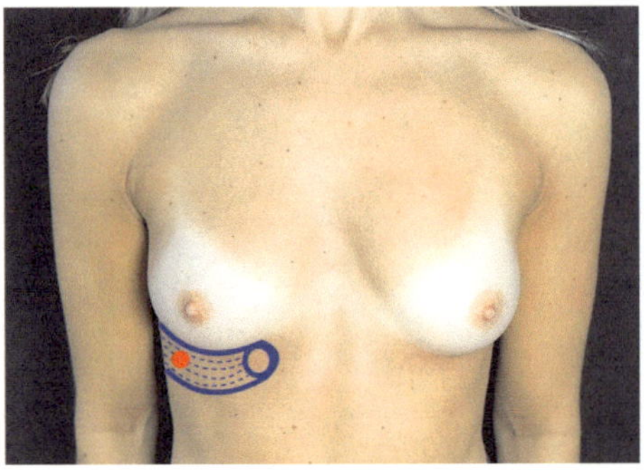

Figure 19.
TYPE III A: Lateral rotation base (based on the LICAP).

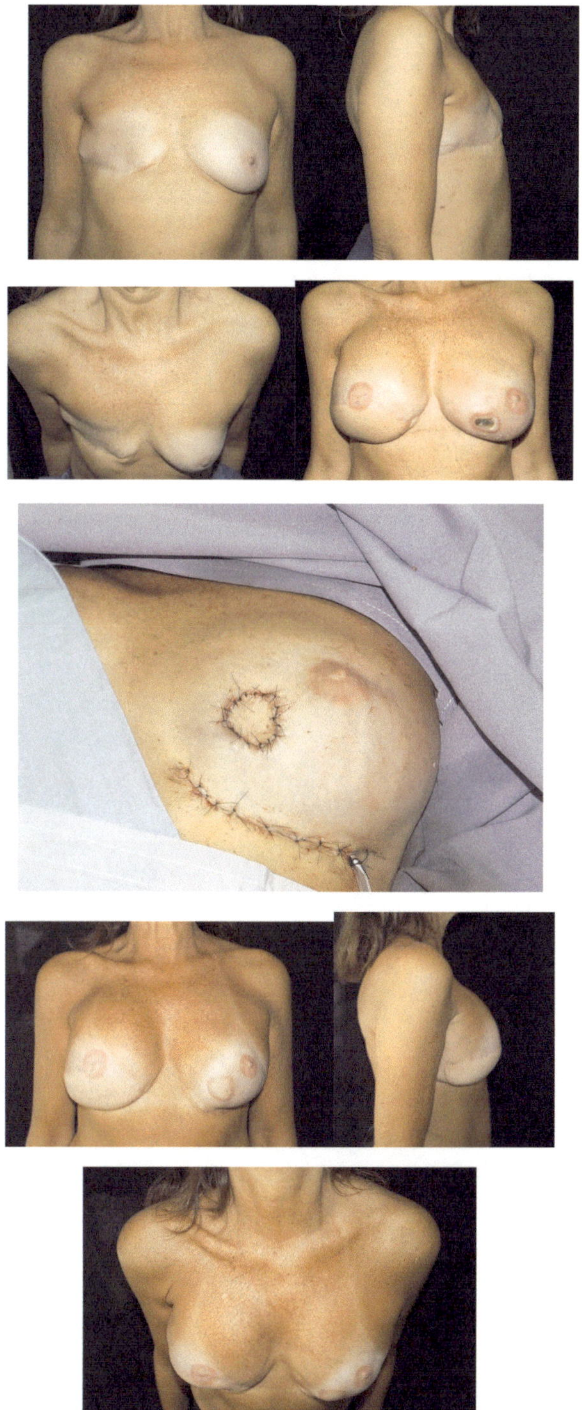

Figure 20.
44-year-old patient with bilateral breast reconstruction. Right breast reconstructed with a latissimus dorsi flap and anatomical breast implant and left risk-reducing mastectomy (RRM). Circumferential necrosis is observed at 6 months in the left breast (the patient applied heat to the area). A type III A flap is placed to cover the localized skin defect. Remote result at 6 months.

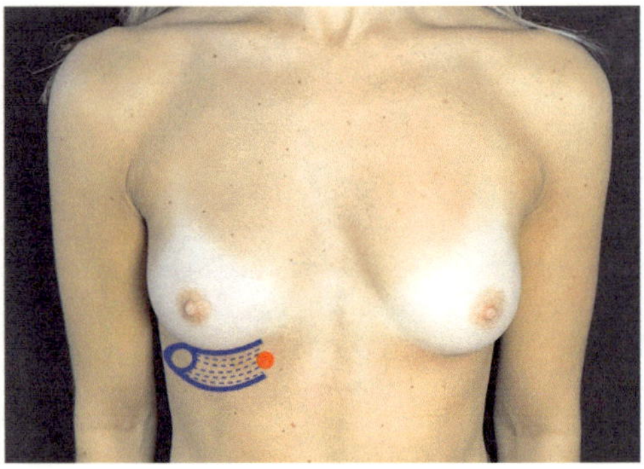

Figure 21.
TYPE III B: Medial rotation base (based on the MICAP).

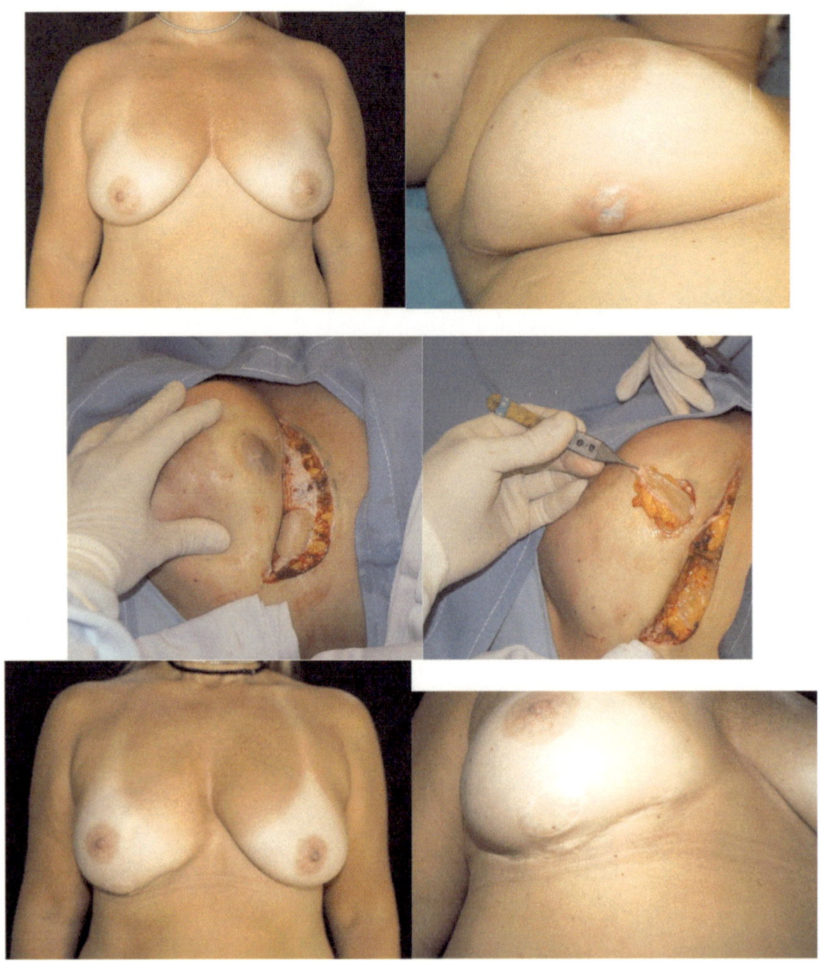

Figure 22.
40-year-old patient with breast reconstruction due to right breast cancer. An area of cutaneous distress is observed in the right breast. Implant close to exposure. A type III B flap is placed on the medial pedicle to cover the localized skin defect. Remote result at 6 months.

The design of the island must be calculated, as well as the length of the flap, which should normally be 5 centimeters longer than the distance between the base and the defect to allow for the resulting bulging of the flap transposition and loss in distance due to rotation.

This flap is very effective in salvaging exposed implants after reconstructive surgery when the area is small and in the lower quadrants.

See **Figure 19**.

See **Figure 20**.

See **Figure 21**.

See **Figure 22**.

6.1.4 TYPE IV: Thoracoabdominal dermofat flaps

The thoracoabdominal dermo-fat flap with a lateral pedicle (Variant IV A) and a medial pedicle (Variant IV B) is a procedure developed by Kijima [14] with a medial pedicle. In the literature, lateral adipose tissue with a medial pedicle in obese patients for bilateral reconstructions is described [15]. The lateral pedicle variant is proposed for selected cases that have correct skin coverage but present esthetic asymmetries with the contralateral breast. It allows greater coverage of the implant and a more natural appearance of the breast. This technique can be complemented with the use of fat grafting (lipofilling), widely used in breast reconstruction to achieve better symmetry, and thus obtain a better esthetic result.

No previous publications have been reported on the use of this lateral pedicle flap. There is a dermo-fat flap in the literature, described for the first time by Rose [16] and later expanded by Irwin et al. [17], to increase the submuscular pocket, thus creating a composite dermal flap, which is sutured to the free edge of the pectoralis major. The authors describe it as a myodermal flap. It consists of the use of de-epithelialized skin from the lower part of the breast.

The adipose tissue is used, as well as the dermis of the upper abdomen to the lateral pedicle to give better thickness to the lower quadrants of the breast. Unlike fat grafting, this procedure is a flap, which ensures greater survival of adipose tissue. It is a simple technique, and when it is performed in selected patients, the resulting scar is cosmetically acceptable.

See **Figure 23**.

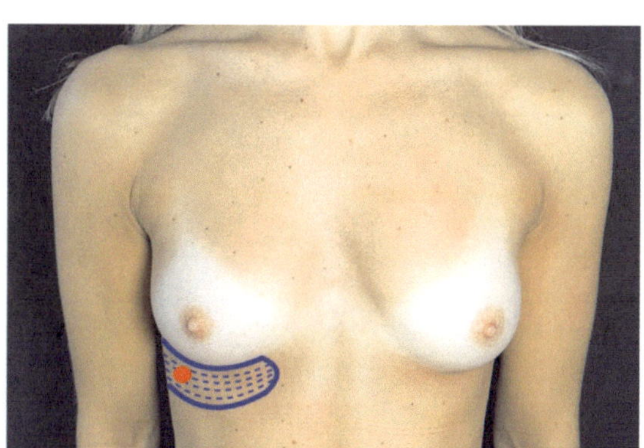

Figure 23.
TYPE IV A: Lateral rotation base (based on the LICAP).

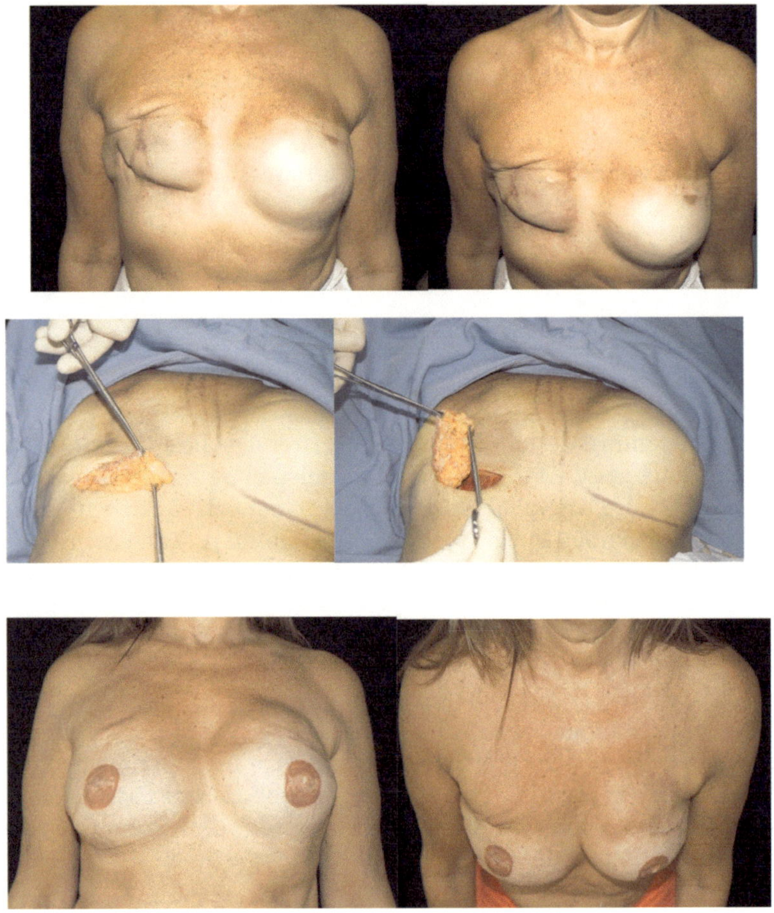

Figure 24.
51-year-old patient with bilateral breast reconstruction. Left mastectomy was performed with immediate implant placement. Right breast underwent risk-reducing mastectomy (RRM). An area of cutaneous suffering is observed in the right complex. Exposure and removal of the implant. A type IV A flap is placed on the lateral pedicle to provide a better cover over the implant to be placed. Remote result at 180 days with the reconstruction of both complexes.

See **Figure 24**.
See **Figure 25**.
See **Figure 26**.

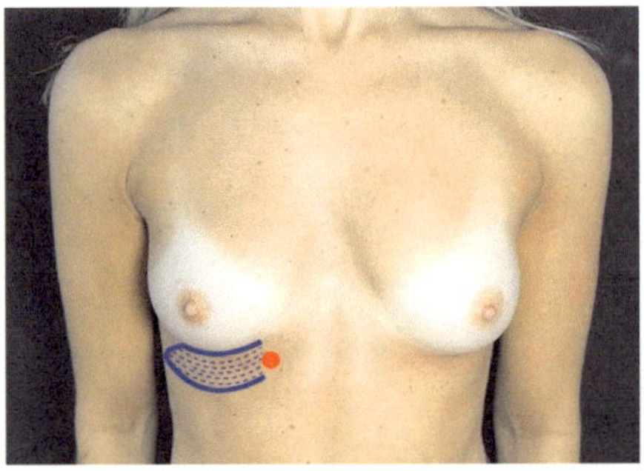

Figure 25.
TYPE IV B: Medial rotation base (based on the MICAP).

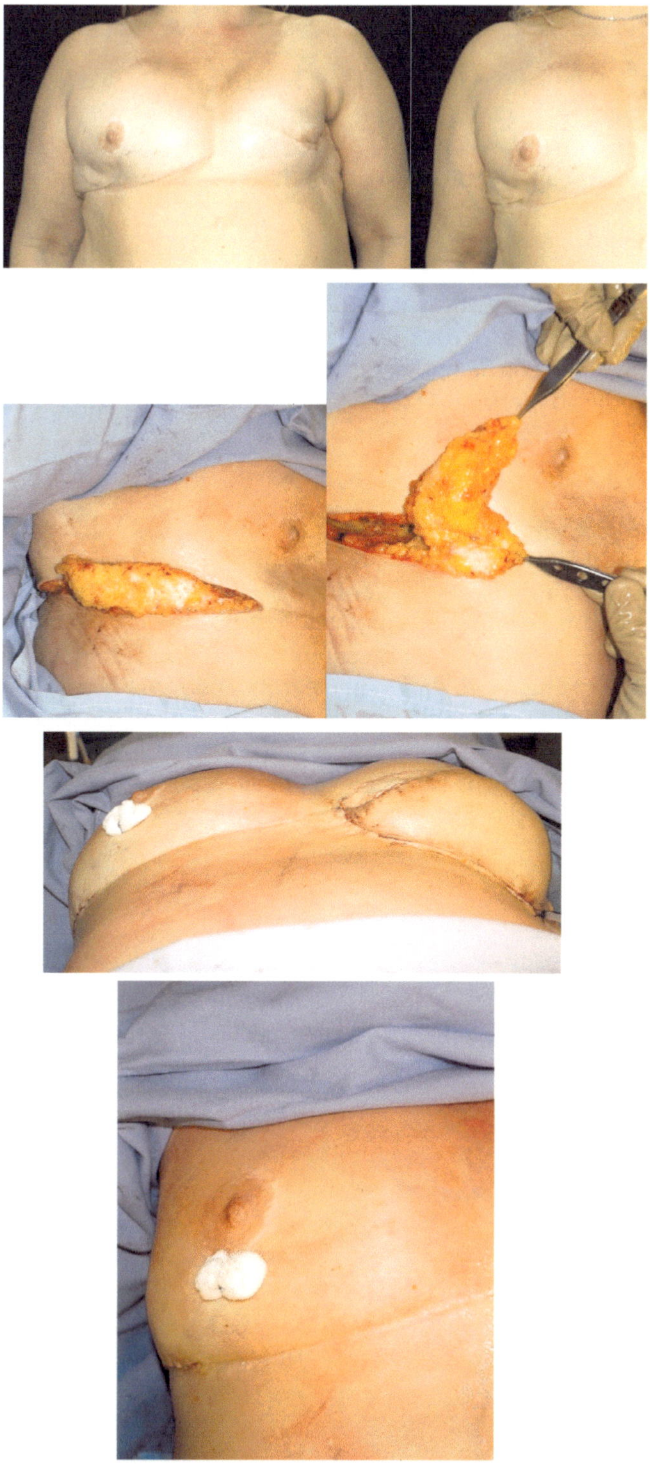

Figure 26.
59-year-old patient with left mastectomy and risk-reducing mastectomy (RRM) in the right breast. A right latissimus dorsi flap and a type IV B left thoracoabdominal flap were made to fill the defect in the lower outer quadrant of the mammary area.

7. Discussion

The thoracoabdominal flaps and variants have been widely used in the field of plastic surgery since, being local flaps, they provide tissue with a similar coloration and texture. They constitute an excellent alternative for the resolution of complications derived from reconstruction surgery with implants since they are remarkably versatile with reliable vasculature, do not involve a sacrifice of muscular structures, and allow an adequate esthetic result [18].

Adequate knowledge of the mechanisms of rotation and sliding of skin tissues is necessary to indicate the use of these types of flaps and to perform them [19, 20]. These flaps make it possible to obtain good results in many patients through a technique that is quick to perform and has a short postoperative stay, especially when compared with other flaps, such as the latissimus dorsi flap or the anterior rectus flap (TRAM, DIEP).

8. Conclusion

The thoracoabdominal flaps are one of the best known and most used flaps when appears a skin necrosis in breast surgery. This publication demonstrates the benefit of using these flaps in complications of breast reconstruction surgeries. A classification is presented to avoid confusion in the nomenclature and two unusual variants of these flaps are exposed (the thoracoabdominal island flap and the thoracoabdominal dermal-fat flap).

The thoracoabdominal flaps have allowed to successfully solve, on numerous occasions, complications that occurred after breast reconstruction.

Conflict of interest

No conflict of interest.

Author details

Ernesto A. Moretti[1,2]

1 Rosario Private Hospital, Rosario, Argentina

2 UAI Medical School, Rosario, Argentina

*Address all correspondence to: doctormorettiuniversidad@gmail.com

IntechOpen

© 2023 The Author(s). Licensee IntechOpen. This chapter is distributed under the terms of the Creative Commons Attribution License (http://creativecommons.org/licenses/by/3.0), which permits unrestricted use, distribution, and reproduction in any medium, provided the original work is properly cited.

References

[1] Woerdeman LA, van Schijndel AW, Hage JJ, et al. Verifying surgical results and risk factors of the lateral thoracodorsal flap. Plastic and Reconstructive Surgery. 2004;**113**:196-203

[2] Spear S. Prophylactic mastectomy and reconstruction: Clinical outcomes and patients satisfaction. Plastic and Reconstructive Surgery. 2008;**2008**:1-9

[3] Holmstrom H, Lossingy C. The lateral thoracodorsal flap in breast reconstruction. Plastic and Reconstructive Surgery. 1986;**77**:933-943

[4] Cronin TD, Upton J, McDonough JM. Reconstruction of the breast after mastectomy. Plastic and Reconstructive Surgery. 1977;**59**:1-14

[5] Bohmert H. Experience in breast reconstruction with thoraco-epigastric and advancement flaps. Acta Chirurgica Belgica. 1980;**79**:105-110

[6] Blomquist L, Malm M. Clinical experience with the lateral thoracodorsal flap in breast reconstruction. Annals of Plastic Surgery. 1999;**43**:7-13

[7] Blomquist L, Malm M, Holmstrom H, Lossingy C. The lateral thoracodorsal flap in breast reconstruction: A comparison between two plastic surgical centers. Scandinavian Journal of Plastic and Reconstructive Surgery. 2000;**34**:331-338

[8] Lossing C, Elander A, Gewalli F. The lateral thoracodorsal flap in breast reconstruction: A long term follow up study. Scandinavian Journal of Plastic and Reconstructive Surgery. 2001;**35**: 183-192

[9] Pontes R, Pontes GH, Serpa NP, Monte AR, Collado CL, Silva FN. Modified lateral thoracodorsal flap: A way out of a difficult problem. Aesthetic Plastic Surgery. 2006;**30**(3):363-368

[10] Carriquiry C, Seoane J, Aycaguer O, Londinsky M. Reconstrucción mamaria con el colgajo toracodorsal de Homstrom: análisis de 6 años de experiencia. Circulation Plastic Iberolatinoam. 2006; **32**(2):83-92

[11] Sastre F, Hernández C, Hayas M, Signes S, Lacorte-Rodés G-M. 20 años de experiencia con el colgajo toracoepigástrico tipo Hölstrom. Circulation Plastic Iberolatinoam. 2008; **34**:211-222

[12] Nebril A, Ramírez B, y col. Colgajos por rotación en la cirugía oncológica de la mama. Fundamentos anatómicos y técnicos para su planificación quirúrgica. Unidad de Mama, Complexo Hospitalario Universitario A Coruña, La Coruña, España. Cirugía Española. 2016; **94**(7):372-378

[13] Rose M, Svensson H. Tunnelled lateral fasciocutaneous thoracodorsal flap with a skin island in breast reconstruction in oncoplastic breast surgery. Journal of Plastic Surgery and Hand Surgery. 2012;**46**:404-409

[14] Kijima Y, Yoshinaka H, Funasako Y, et al. Immediate reconstruction using thoracodorsal adipofascial flap after partial mastectomy. Breast. 2009;**18**:126-129

[15] Shin J, Park E, Kim Y, Nam S. The lateral thoracodorsal flap in delayed bilateral breast reconstruction for an obese patient with redundant lateral Chest Wall soft tissue. Archieves of Aesthetic Plastic Surgery. 2015;**21**(1):26-29

[16] Ross GL. One stage breast reconstruction following prophylactic

mastectomy for ptotic breasts: The inferior dermal flap and implant. Journal of Plastic, Reconstructive & Aesthetic Surgery. 2012;**65**(9):1204e8

[17] Irwin G, Black A, Refsum S, McIntosh S. Skin-reducing mastectomy and one-stage implant reconstruction with a myodernal flap: A safe and effective technique in risk reducing and therapeutic mastectomy. Journal of Plastic, Reconstructive & Aesthetic Surgery. 2013;**66**:1188-1194

[18] De Weerd L, Woerdeman LA, Hage JJ. The lateral thoracodorsal flap as a salvage procedure for partial transverse rectus abdominis myocutaneous or deep inferior epigastric perforator flap loss in breast reconstruction. Annals of Plastic Surgery. 2005;**54**:590-594

[19] Munhoz AM, Montag E, Arruda EG, Aldrighi C, Gemperli R, Aldrighi JM, et al. The role of the lateral thoracodorsal fasciocutaneous flap in immediate conservative breast surgery reconstruction. Plastic Reconstruction Surgery. 2006;**117**(6):1699-1710

[20] Elzawawy E, Kelada M, Al Karmouty A. New possible surgical approaches for the submammary Adipofascial flap based on its arterial supply. Anatomy Research International. 2016;**2016**:7696010

Chapter 7

Flaps for Breast Reconstruction

Raj Manas and Dhanushya Gohil

Abstract

Breast is one important organ of women that not only has functional importance of lactation, but also defines the femininity of a woman. Any lass of breast either partial or total may cause psychosocial impact on women's life. Thus, in case of loss due to various reasons, plastic surgeons involved in oncosurgery team should offer reconstruction to restore breast volume, size, and self-esteem of patients. The chapter aims to describe the various deformities of the breast following cancer, trauma, burn, and reconstructive options in terms of flaps. The various flaps described for breast reconstruction are LD flap, TRAM flap, DIEP flap, and expander implant techniques. The readers will be able to execute the planning for breast reconstruction knowing the indications and contraindications of using a particular flap, surgical techniques of flap elevations, and post-operative care and management.

Keywords: breast reconstruction, flaps for breast reconstruction, mastectomy, LD flap, TRAM flap, DIEP flap

1. Introduction

The breast is a vital organ of women which not only has functional importance but also provides femininity to the individual. Loss of breasts following mastectomy especially post cancer affects women's health functionally and psychologically. Apart from cancer, the breast can also be scarred, or affected partially or totally in case of burn or trauma. Every effort should be made to offer reconstruction in mastectomy or patients with breast deformities.

The various options described for breast reconstruction are LD (latissimus dorsi) flap, TRAM (Transverse rectus abdominis myo-cutaneous) flap, DIEAP (Deep inferior epigastric artery perforator) flap, and expander implant techniques. With the advancement in microsurgery, the free flaps have become the gold standard in breast reconstruction. Before planning the reconstruction of the breast, reconstructive surgeons should examine the patient as a whole, discuss the various options with advantages and disadvantages of each technique, and offer a complete reconstruction including breast mound and nipple-areola reconstruction to the patients. The same should be discussed with oncosurgeons regarding the staging of disease and the extent of resection of diseased parts.

We have aimed to provide an overview of all options available for breast reconstruction so that readers will be able to execute the planning for breast reconstruction knowing the indications and contraindications of using a particular flap, surgical techniques of flap elevations, and post-operative care and management.

IntechOpen

2. Latissimus Dorsi myo-cutaneous flap

Introduction: Latissimus Dorsi or LD myocutenous flap was initially described by Ignio Tansini in 1906 [1]. Being a regional flap with a reliable blood supply makes it a good option for breast reconstruction especially for women with small size breasts. However, it is often used along with implants or prostheses so it is not preferred as a first choice by many surgeons.

2.1 Relevant anatomy

Latissimus Dorsi is the largest, fan-shaped, flat muscle situated on the back on both sides which *arises from* the lower 6th ribs, spinous process of 6th or 7th thoracic vertebrae to 5th lumbar vertebrae, from sacrum, posterior iliac crest, and thoraco-lumbar fascia, and gets *inserted at* the bicipital groove of the humerus. It is *supplied by* the thoracodorsal artery and vein which is a branch of the subscapular artery and vein respectively and *innervated by* the thoracodorsal nerve. It also has several minor pedicles, that arise from perforators of the intercostal artery, thus making it the *type V muscle* type of Mathes and Nahai. The main *function* of the LD muscle is extension, adduction, and internal rotation of the arm.

2.2 Flap harvesting

Marking (**Figure 1**): Marking of the flap is preferred in a standing position. The midline of the back is marked which is the posterior border of LD. Then posterior axillary line, which runs from the posterior border of the axilla to the iliac crest

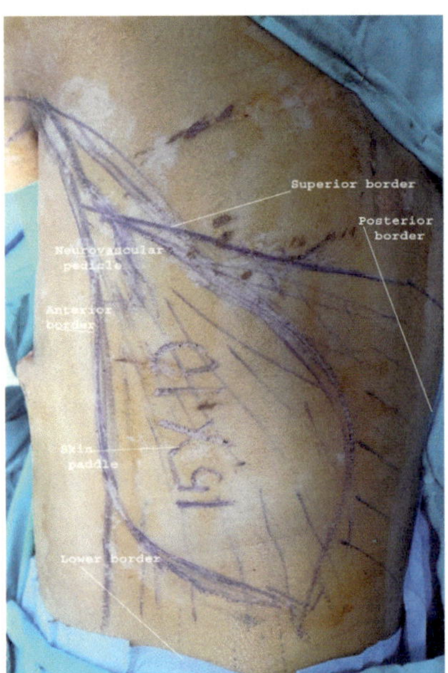

Figure 1.
Marking for LD myo-cutaneous flap.

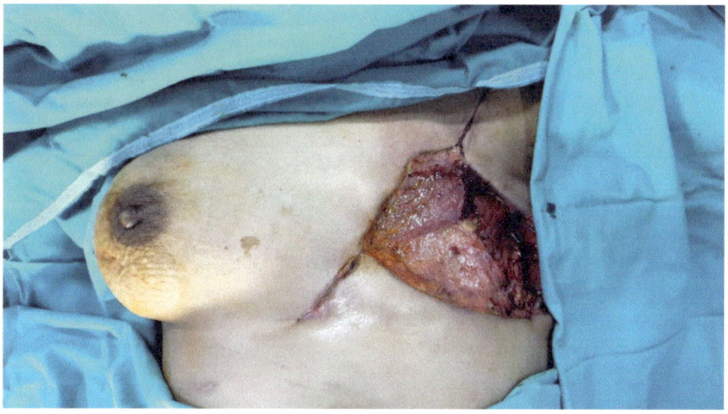

Figure 2.
Defect after mastectomy on left side.

corresponds to the anterior border. A line joining from the midline touches the inferior angle of the scapula and joins the posterior axillary fold is the superior border. The Iliac crest is considered an inferior border of muscle [2].

Once all four borders are marked, the skin paddle is marked which can be drawn obliquely, or transverse according to defect size (**Figure 2**) and surgeon's preference with an aim of closure of donor area primarily and scar to be hidden maximally. Hammond recommends designing a skin paddle along the RSTL (relaxed skin tension line) [2]. The pedicle of LD, the thoracodorsal vessels is marked which is 2 cm behind and parallel to the anterior border of the muscle and 10–12 cm below the axillary fold.

Positioning: It is preferred to harvest LD myo-cutaneous flap in a lateral position with the arm abducted to 90 degrees, medially rotated, extended and supported on the other side by arm support. One should also never forget to put cotton or a pad over the bony prominence of the opposite shoulder and between knees to avoid any pressure necrosis due to prolonged operating time.

Technique: Once skin paddle and incisions are marked, it is begun with infiltration of tumescent solution or adrenaline with saline (1:2 lakh ratio) along the proposed incision to reduce bleeding. An incision is made over the margin of the marked skin paddle and LD muscle with a layer of fat over it is exposed from all sides. Fat provides a bit of bulk for breast reconstruction. However, for free flap or when it is used for another region, it is ideal to harvest the muscle only. Once the muscle is exposed, the anterior border of LD muscle is delineated and dissected which lies along the anterior axillary line. By doing a blunt dissection, a few centimeters behind the anterior border, the neurovascular pedicle of the LD muscle can be easily seen lying just below the muscle. Once the pedicle is seen, the muscle is dissected and cut from below at the thoracolumbar fascia. We can easily identify and define a thin layer of fat between LD and underlying intercostal muscles. If we stay in the fat layer, there is less chance of bleeding. Also, it is important to cauterize several perforators arising from the lumbar artery and intercostal artery to secure hemostasis.

Once the muscle is cut from its inferior and posterior border, it is dissected upward. At the inferior angle of the scapula, there is an intermingling of muscle fibers with teres major. The muscle is further dissected incorporating the vascular and neural pedicle and the flap is harvested (**Figure 3**). A tunnel is created from the defect through the axilla and muscle with a skin paddle is retrieved through the tunnel. During tunneling it is

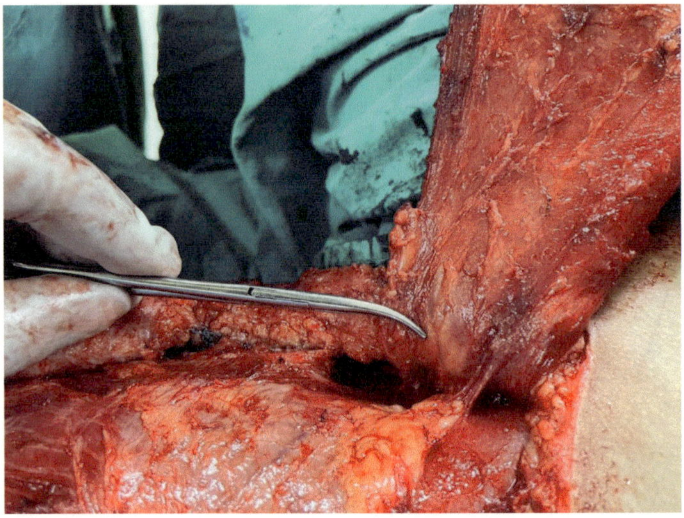

Figure 3.
Neurovascular pedicle of LD flap.

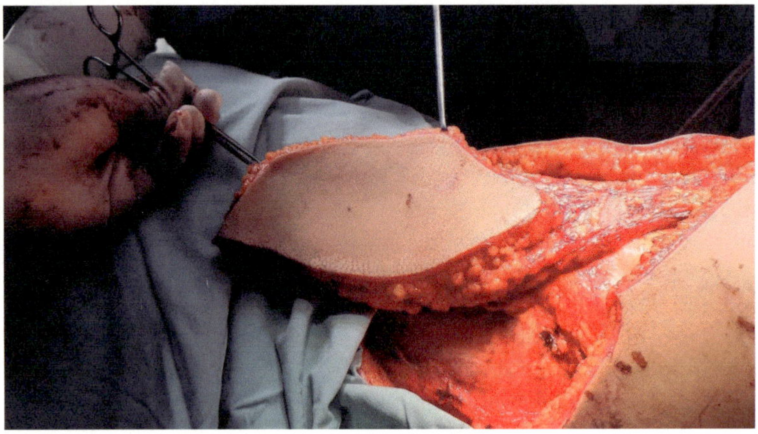

Figure 4.
Harvested LD myo-cutaneous flap attached with pedicle.

always preferred to create a wide tunnel at least two to three fingers width wide to avoid compression of muscle and pedicle. If there is difficult reach, the muscle can be detached from its insertion and the flap is islanded over the pedicle (**Figure 4**). The flap is inset (**Figure 5**). A drain is always placed at the donor as well as the recipient site. To avoid hematoma, one can put several quilting sutures from under the skin to the back muscles. A compression dressing is provided in the form of dynaplast.

2.3 Complications

- Hematoma and seroma are the most common complications, so the drain should be removed only when it is less than 10–20 ml.
- Partial or total flap necrosis may occur

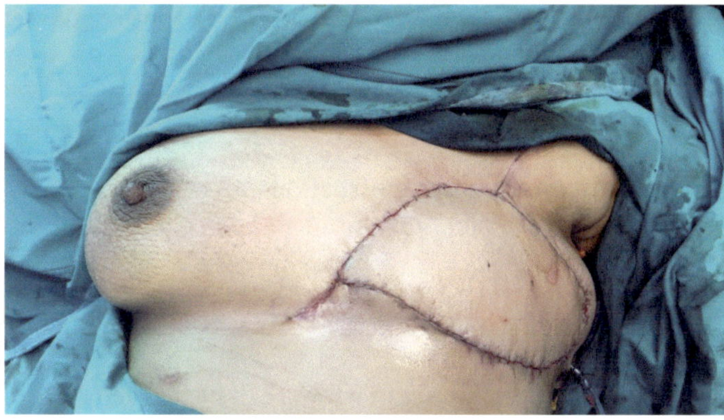

Figure 5.
LD flap after inset at the mastectomy site.

- Donor site scar may pose a problem especially if a large skin paddle was taken.

2.4 Contraindication

- Previous thoracotomy or injury to the neurovascular pedicle of LD muscle
- When a large amount of the breast is required
- Not suitable for thin patients as it may not provide bulk to the reconstructed breast

3. Rectus abdominis myo-cutaneous flap

Introduction: Rectus abdominis muscle can be harvested along with skin and subcutaneous tissue; either pedicle or free flap; either vertically oriented (VRAM) or transverse (TRAM) or either superiorly based or inferiorly based. The transverse rectus abdominis muscle (TRAM) flap became popular because of its obvious low donor site morbidity and lower abdominal tissue to be excised during abdominoplasty operation. TRAM flap was evolved in 1982 by Hartrampf as part of an abdomino-plasty operation where the pannus is usually discarded but can be utilized for breast reconstruction preserving its blood supply and one rectus abdominis muscle [3].

3.1 Applied anatomy

Rectus abdominis is a *vertically oriented* flat muscle *situated on* the bilateral side of the midline of the abdomen and en-sheathed into the anterior and posterior rectus sheath. It *arises* from the costochondral parts of the 5th, 6th, and 7th ribs and xiphi-sternum and is *inserted* into pubic symphysis. It has two dominant vascular pedicles, thus making it a kind of *type III* muscle. Superiorly it is *nourished by* the superior epi-gastric artery and veins that arise from internal mammary arteries and veins respec-tively and inferiorly it is supplied by the deep inferior epigastric artery and veins which is a branch of the external iliac artery and accompanying veins respectively. It is also supplied by several minor pedicles of subcostal and intercostal arteries and veins.

Based on the arterial and venous circulation pattern, the lower abdomen is divided into four zones (I–IV) of perfusion. *Zone I* is just above the muscle on the ipsilateral side, and *Zone II* is the zone opposite to the muscle on the contralateral side. *Zone III* is the ipsilateral side adjacent to Zone I and *Zone IV* is the contralateral side adjacent to Zone II.

The anterior rectus sheath overlies the rectus abdominis muscle and the anterior rectus sheath contains three tendinous intersections, first at the level of costal cartilage, second at the midpoint between the umbilicus and costal cartilage, and third at the level of umbilicus.

3.2 Flap harvesting

Flap marking: **(Figure 6)** The flap's skin paddle can be marked *vertically* along the muscle or *transversely* in the lower abdomen. In the case of women with pannus who desire to undergo abdominoplasty surgery, the flap is marked in the same fashion as an abdominoplasty incision. Lower abdominal tissue is pinched with the thumb and index finger and that determines the donor area to be closed primarily. The both sides of ASIS (Anterior superior iliac spine) are marked, then an incision is marked joining the two ASIS meeting in the midline just above the mons pubis. Another curvilinear incision is marked superiorly so the skin paddle of the flap becomes boat-shaped or elliptical. Both sides of muscles are marked along with two subcostal sides. The umbilicus is marked circumferentially for dissection. It is also important to examine the presence of rectus diastasis (straight leg raising test) which is marked accordingly.

Technique: An incision is made first in the lower part, and skin and subcutaneous tissue are incised. If possible, an attempt may be made to dissect the superficial inferior epigastric veins which will be in the subcutaneous space of the lower abdomen on

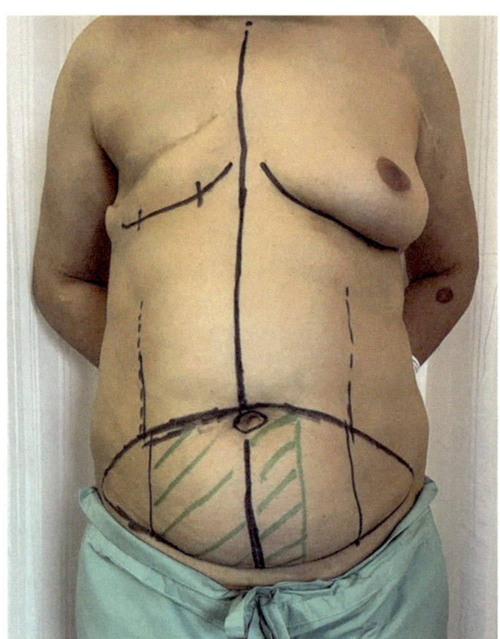

Figure 6.
Marking for TRAM flap.

both sides. The same vein can be used for supercharging in case of venous congestion of superiorly based pedicle flap or as an extra draining vein for free flap. The superior incision is made and the elliptical flap is elevated from lateral to medial. Once we reach near the lateral border of the anterior rectus sheath, we get the lateral row of perforators, that is cauterized and sacrificed. Anterior rectus sheath is incised and a plane is dissected between the rectus muscle anteriorly and posteriorly, away from the skin paddle. It is important to maintain the continuity of the rectus sheath anteriorly with the skin paddle and muscles. Also, the tendinous intersection found at three defined levels needs to be dissected. In case of *superiorly based pedicle flap*, the superior pedicle is dissected which lies in the subcostal region deep to muscle in its medial half. The muscle including soft tissue is dissected from below upwards and is brought over the defects for insetting. A tunnel is created between the defect and the origin the of muscle (**Figure 7**). The inset is completed.

For raising it as a free flap for breast reconstruction, it can be as VRAM or TRAM. The commonly performed TRAM has its pedicle in the lower part, once we elevate the muscle, it is easier to identify the pedicle which is dissected to its origins. It is usually found lateral half of the muscle in the lower parts. The muscle is cut superiorly and the flap includes skin and a subcutaneous tissue along with muscle. We can reconstruct the breast by providing the good bulk of muscle by either pedicle or free rectus abdominis myocutenous flap (**Figure 8**).

The donor area: The donor area is closed primarily in layers after securing the hemostasis. If there is a presence of rectus diastasis, rectus plication can be done. Also, any hernial orifices can be reduced and repaired in the same sitting by putting mesh. It can be combined with the dissection of upper abdominal tissue along with the repositioning of the umbilicus.

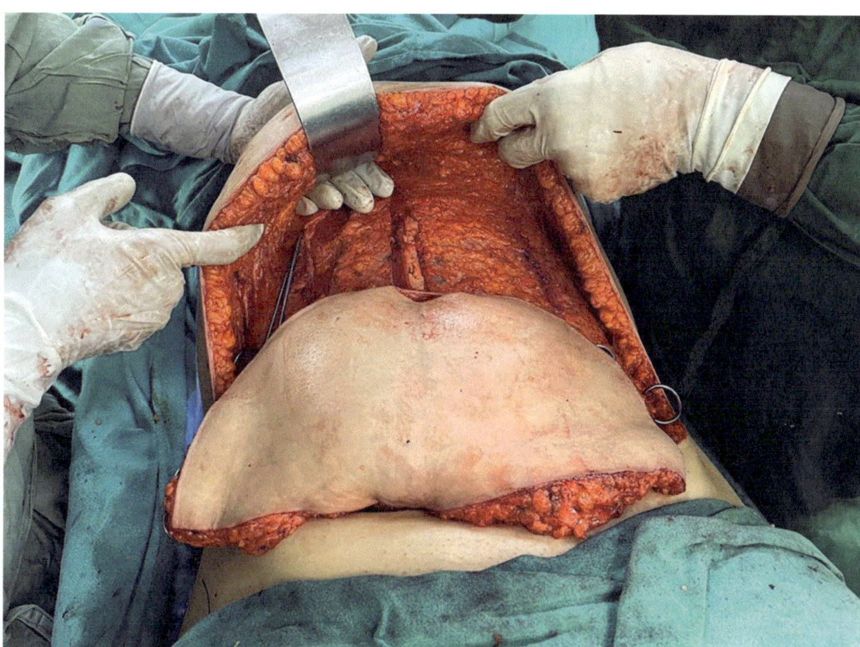

Figure 7.
TRAM flap dissected with the creation of tunnel through mastectomy side.

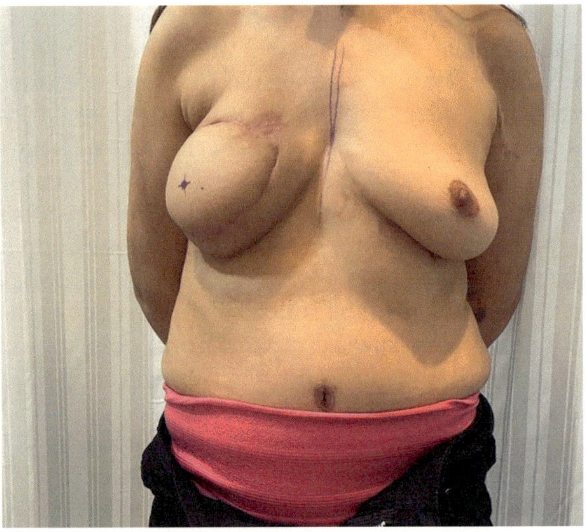

Figure 8.
Late post-operative result of TRAM flap reconstruction.

3.3 Complications

- Partial or total flap necrosis
- Fat necrosis
- Incisional hernia at the donor site
- Wound dehiscence

4. Deep inferior epigastric artery perforator flap

Deep Inferior Epigastric Artery Perforator or DIEAP flap is currently one of the most popular flaps used for breast reconstruction because of the obvious reason of minimum donor site morbidity (being muscle sparing) compared to TRAM flap and with less complication rate like incisional hernia and fat necrosis.

4.1 Applied anatomy

DIEAP flap is based on musculocutaneous perforators arising from the deep inferior epigastric artery. The regional vascular anatomy of the DIEAP flap is the same as the TRAM flap except one should be familiar with the location and course of the perforators to be dissected both anatomically and surgically. As abdominal wall is nourished by two epigastric arterial systems. The superior epigastric arises from the internal mammary artery and the deep inferior epigastric artery arises from the external iliac artery. After originating from an external iliac artery, it runs upwards and medially and goes behind the posterior rectus sheath where it runs intramuscularly and gives two branches. These branches run intramuscularly and then anastomoses with arcades of various vessels at the subdermal level. These myo-cutaneous perforators apart from the muscle route, can directly supply to the skin also. Once traversing through the muscle, these perforators further pierce the anterior rectus sheath and then supply the subcutaneous tissue and skin. Most of these perforators are found around the umbilicus and in the medial and middle 1/3rd of the muscle [4].

4.2 Flap harvesting

Pre-operative considerations: It is important to evaluate the patient as a whole. Any comorbid conditions and history of smoking should be evaluated and smoking should be stopped at least 3 weeks before surgery. Also, any previous abdominal surgeries like abdominoplasty, liposuction, or Caesarian section scar are not a good candidate for DIEP flap reconstruction. The defect size and volume is assessed comparing with contra-lateral side (**Figure 9**).

Pre-operative mapping of perforators: Although there are several tools like handheld Doppler, color Doppler scan, and contrast-enhanced CT scan. The current investigation of choice is HRCT angiography which determines the location and size of perforators along with their branching pattern.

Marking: The marking of the DIEAP flap is the same as the TRAM flap or abdominoplasty incision with an additional marking for perforators. A boat-shaped or elliptical incision is marked joining the two sides ASIS, umbilicus, and mons pubis (**Figure 10**).

Positioning: The patient is in a supine position with the arm abducted and supported on both sides over the armrest.

Technique: In general, the lower border of an ellipse is incised first and subcutaneous tissue is dissected with dissection of the superficial inferior epigastric vein on both sides. These veins can be utilized for supercharging the flap in case of venous compromise. The next step is the identification of perforators of the deep inferior epigastric artery. One can dissect both sides of perforators and choose the suitable one. For that one side is dissected first and the other side is preserved in case of non-availability or reduced size and pulsation of perforators. The circumferential incision along the umbilicus is made and the superior incision is completed by doing careful dissection around the umbilicus pedicle. The deep fascia is identified initially from the superior incision and then dissected from lateral to medial. The perforators start

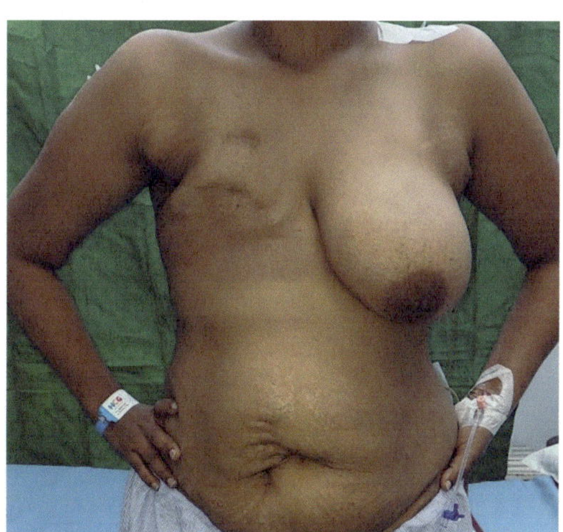

Figure 9.
Pre-operating defect after mastectomy (for secondary reconstruction).

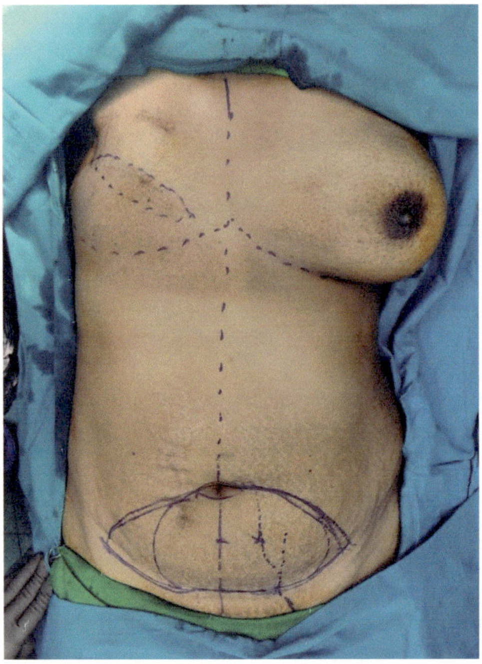

Figure 10.
Marking for DIEAP flap.

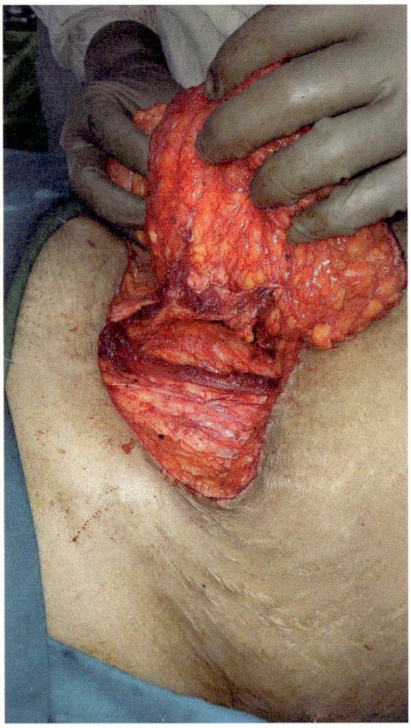

Figure 11.
Dissection of perforators of DIEAP flap.

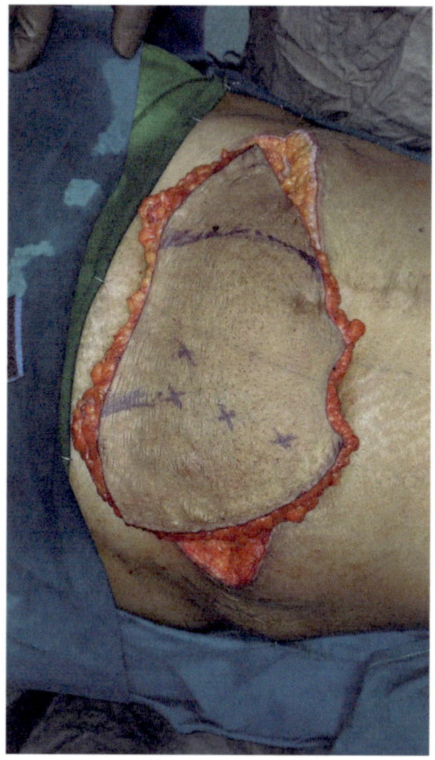

Figure 12.
Harvested DIEAP flap.

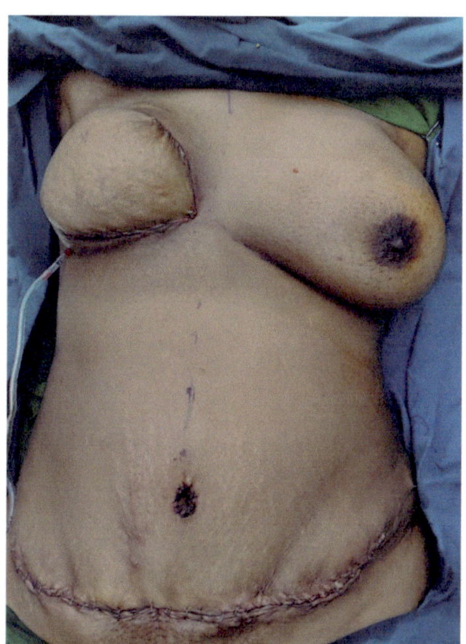

Figure 13.
Immediate post-operative result after insetting on table.

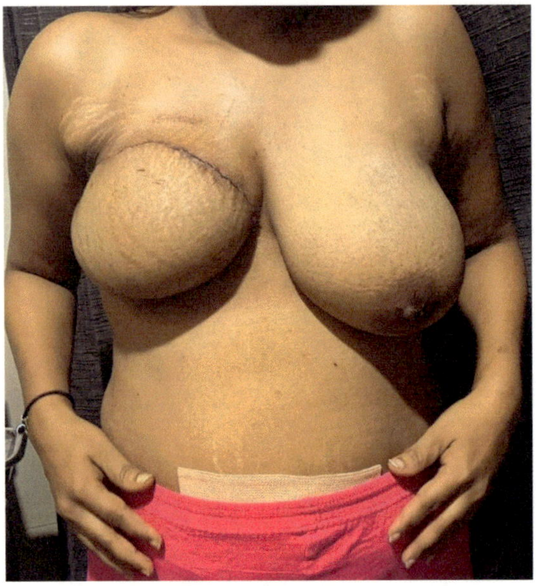

Figure 14.
Post-operative result.

from the lateral border of the rectus sheath. We try to dissect all perforators that come in the way or are predefined by radiological imaging and an appropriate perforator is chosen with adequate diameter and pulsation. The perforators are dissected till it pierce the anterior rectus sheath. A longitudinal (**Figure 11**) incision is made into the anterior rectus sheath and the perforator is further dissected en route to rectus muscle whether it further goes through the posterior rectus sheath. The perforator is dissected from its origin of the deep inferior epigastric artery which is further dissected till its origin inferno-medially (**Figure 12**) from the external iliac artery and the flap is islanded and harvested with its pedicle. Zone IV of perfusion is usually discarded and the flap is inset at the recipient site and followed by anastomosis.

The donor area (**Figure 13**) is closed primarily. In case of difficult approximation, the superior part of the abdominal flap is dissected in the midline and a neo-position of the umbilicus is created. The rectus sheath is repaired with a braided ethibond suture. The drains are kept in situ. DIEAP flap can provide a good volume without any donor site morbidity (**Figure 14**).

4.3 Complications

Partial and total flap failure.
Wound dehiscence at the donor area.

5. Other flaps and techniques

5.1 PAP flap

The first live demonstration of PAP flap was by Allen in 2010. PAP flap named as profunda artery perforator flap was originally described for breast reconstruction.

It is based on perforators of the profunda femoris artery which traverses the adductor magnus muscle and supplies the medial and posterior side of the thigh. This can be considered a good option for breast reconstruction when abdominal skin is unavailable and a DIEAP flap is not possible [5].

5.2 TDAP flap

TDAP or Thoracodorsal artery perforator flap is based on perforators of the thoracodorsal artery. It was first described by Angrigiani in 1992 since then it has been a good source of regional tissue for partial or total breast reconstruction [6]. Being a local or regional flap, it can provide the best color and texture to match the breast. However, it has been used mainly for small defects. Ebraheim and Manas have described using it for post-burn breast contracture especially inferior pole contracture with excellent results and they recommend using more bulky tissue for reconstruction after the recreated defect of grade III breast contracture as TDAP alone will be insufficient [7].

5.3 Gluteal artery perforator flap

It consists of two flaps named superior gluteal artery perforator flap and inferior gluteal artery perforator flap. The SGAP flap or superior artery perforator flap is based on perforators of the superior gluteal artery which is a branch of the internal iliac artery, the flap was originally described in 1993 and has been a good option for breast reconstruction due to minimum donor site morbidities.

The same group described the inferior gluteal artery perforator flap in 2004. Based on perforators of the inferior gluteal artery, a branch of the anterior division of the internal iliac artery that supply that supplies the skin in the lower part of the gluteal region or inferior gluteal crease [8]. However, the inferior gluteal artery perforator flap is less preferred because of an obvious scar over which the patient sits and the risk of injury to the sciatic nerve.

5.4 Fat grafting

Fat grafting is one of the good options with no or minimum donor site morbidity at various stages of reconstruction. Autologous fat grafting serves as an adjunct to not only implant-based and autologous reconstruction but also a good option in primary defects following mastectomy in some selective patients as described by Turner et al. [9]. The only disadvantage with fat grafting is that fat may get absorbed over a period of time and may require multiple settings to achieve a desirable outcome.

5.5 Nipple-areola complex reconstruction

The various technique described for nipple reconstruction includes nipple sharing, various local flaps like skate flaps, dermal fat flap, and star flap, etc. described by various authors along with autologous cartilage graft or implant-based prosthesis. For the areola, a graft from the opposite areola, labia majora, or tattooing is preferred [10].

5.6 Management of contra-lateral breast for bilateral symmetry

In level II oncoplastic breast surgery where there is 20–50% excision of breast parenchymal tissue and the resultant defect cannot be reconstructed with either tissue displacement or replacement technique (flap) with symmetry to other breast; such cases require reduction mammoplasty for contralateral breast. Breast reduction to bring symmetry to both breasts can be done immediately at the time of oncoplastic breast surgery or after completion of chemo-radiation. However, if patients do not want to undergo any procedures on the normal side, a small volume of fat can be injected on the reconstructed side to bring symmetry to some extent [11].

6. Conclusion

Breast reconstruction is a challenging task with a number of options available for reconstruction. Each option should be brief to the patients with its pros and cons and should be chosen based on defect size, the types of mastectomy, availability of donor site, symmetry with opposite breast, patient's medical history and surgeon's skill (**Algorithm 1**).

Algorithm 1. Algorithm of breast reconstruction.

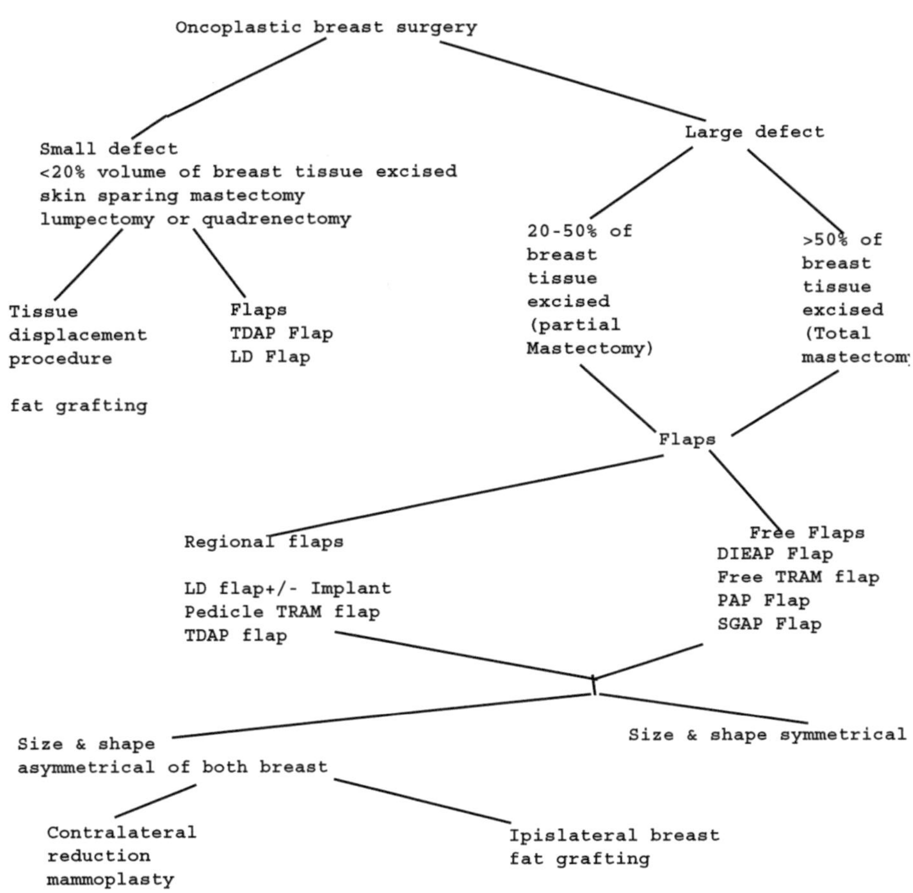

Author details

Raj Manas[1]* and Dhanushya Gohil[2]

1 All India Institute of Medical Sciences, New Delhi, India

2 HCG Cancer Center, Ahmedabad, India

*Address all correspondence to: rajmanas007@rediffmail.com

IntechOpen

© 2023 The Author(s). Licensee IntechOpen. This chapter is distributed under the terms of the Creative Commons Attribution License (http://creativecommons.org/licenses/by/3.0), which permits unrestricted use, distribution, and reproduction in any medium, provided the original work is properly cited.

References

[1] Ribuffo D, Cigna E, Gerald GL, et al. Iginio Tansini revisited. European Review for Medical and Pharmacological Sciences. 2015;**19**(13):2477-2481

[2] Hammond DC. Latissimus dorsi flap breast reconstruction. Clinics in Plastic Surgery. 2007;**34**(1):75-vii. DOI: 10.1016/j.cps.2006.11.008

[3] Hartrampf CR, Scheflan M, Black PW. Breast reconstruction with a transverse abdominal island flap. Plastic and Reconstructive Surgery. 1982;**69**(2):216-225. DOI: 10.1097/00006534-198202000-00006

[4] Gagnon AR, Blondeel PN. Deep and superficial inferior epigastric artery perforator flaps. In: Wei FC, Mardini S, editors. Flaps and Reconstructive Surgery. Philadelphia, PA: Elsevier; 2009. pp. 501-522

[5] Lu J, Zhang KK, Graziano FD, Nelson JA, Allen RJ Jr. Alternative donor sites in autologous breast reconstruction: A clinical practice review of the PAP flap. Gland Surgery. 2023;**12**(4):516-526. DOI: 10.21037/gs-22-603

[6] Angrigiani C, Rancati A, Escudero E, Artero G, Gercovich G, Deza EG. Propeller thoracodorsal artery perforator flap for breast reconstruction [published correction appears in Gland Surg. 2017 Dec;6(6):753]. Gland Surgery. 2014;**3**(3):174-180. DOI: 10.3978/j.issn.2227-684X.2014.06.04

[7] Ebrahiem AA, Manas RK. Inferior pole breast reconstruction by TDAP flap in post-burn breast contracture. European Journal of Plastic Surgery. 2019;**42**:337-342. DOI: 10.1007/s00238-019-1504-x

[8] Allen RJ, Soueid NE, Vasile J, Mountcastle TS, Chiu ES, Levine JL. Superior and inferior gluteal artery perforator flaps. In: Wei FC, Mardini S, editors. Flaps and Reconstructive Surgery. Philadelphia, PA: Elsevier; 2009. pp. 523-537

[9] Turner A, Abu-Ghname A, Davis MJ, Winocour SJ, Hanson SE, Chu CK. Fat grafting in breast reconstruction. Seminars in Plastic Surgery. 2020;**34**(1):17-23. DOI: 10.1055/s-0039-1700959. Epub 2020 February 15

[10] Paolini G, Firmani G, Briganti F, Sorotos M, Santanelli di Pompeo F. Guiding nipple-areola complex reconstruction: Literature review and proposal of a new decision-making algorithm. Aesthetic Plastic Surgery. 2021;**45**(3):933-945. DOI: 10.1007/s00266-020-02047-9. Epub 2020 November 20

[11] Kaviani AMD, Safavi AMD, Mirsharifi RMD. Immediate and delayed contralateral symmetrization in oncoplastic breast reduction: Patients' choices and technique formulation. Plastic and Reconstructive Surgery – Global Open. 2015;**3**(1):e286. DOI: 10.1097/GOX.0000000000000246

Chapter 8

Alternative Flap-Based Breast Reconstruction: The PAP Flap

Michael Borrero, Robert Allen and Hugo St. Hilaire

Abstract

The profunda artery perforator flap, like many perforator-based flaps in breast reconstruction, has evolved from its initial introduction more than a decade ago. It is considered by many to be the priority alternative flap when abdominal flaps are unavailable. Several configurations of the flap may be utilized routinely, making this flap particularly versatile for mild-moderate volume breast reconstruction. Additionally, as reconstructive microsurgeons become more adept, they strive to achieve an esthetically pleasing breast in the first stage. The PAP flap is particularly suited for this endeavor, as its ability to be contoured to simulate a natural breast mound at time of inset is impressive.

Keywords: profunda artery perforator flap, PAP flap, autologous breast reconstruction, thigh flap, flap contouring

1. Introduction

Breast reconstruction by way of the profunda artery perforator flap, also known as the PAP flap, came to fruition in 2010. Historically, this free flap is the culmination of advancements dating back to the myocutaneous posterior thigh flap introduced by Hurwitz and Walton in 1980 [1, 2]. Subsequently, the flap was modified by Angrigiani et al. [3] and Song et al. [2] within the realm of pressure ulcer and lower extremity reconstruction.

Later, Dr. Robert Allen pioneered its use in breast reconstruction in Mexico City in 2010. He designed the flap off the first or second perforator from the profunda artery in an ellipse that extended from an anterior point at the origin of the adductor longus, to a posterior point at the end of the inferior gluteal crease [4, 5]. This would be colloquially known as the transverse PAP flap.

This flap added to the ever-growing repertoire of the reconstructive microsurgeon; specifically, it offered a perforator-based flap from the lower extremity. This was exceedingly beneficial when the abdomen, undoubtedly the most useful donor site, was unavailable for reconstructive efforts. Advantages of the PAP flap became readily apparent—good donor site location with minimal morbidity, consistent and reliable vascular anatomy, adequate pedicle length and caliber, ability to harvest from supine position—however there are drawbacks when compared to alternatives, primarily the lack of volume [4, 6]. Modern advancements in the flap, however, counter this disadvantage, especially when considering the relatively novel 'fleur-de-PAP', as well as stacked flap procedures. This chapter explores the fundamentals of PAP flap breast reconstruction.

2. Patient selection and considerations

Breast reconstruction begins at the initial consultation with patient selection and surgical planning. Modern advancements in microsurgical techniques created an impetus for innovative flap design. This includes the PAP flap, which has become our preferred alternative donor site secondary only to the abdomen. With thorough understanding of outcomes over the past decade, we have become more proficient in restoring native breast volume and esthetic contour at the first stage. When considering any patient for microsurgical breast reconstruction, a thorough history and physical exam is invaluable. Paying particular attention to body habitus and subcutaneous volume distribution of the abdomen and thighs is critical to achieving an optimal result. The indications for using PAP flaps are essentially contraindications to using the abdomen as a donor site. The only conceivable contraindication to harvesting a PAP flap is lack of perforator presence, most likely due to trauma or previous surgery (e.g. medial thigh lift).

The ideal candidate for PAP flap reconstruction is a breast with mild to moderate volume. The ideal body habitus is one who carries excess subcutaneous tissue in the hips and thighs more so than the abdomen, what is colloquially known as being "pear-shaped". In our experience a single component PAP flap weighs on average between 250 to 450 grams, depending on the quality of tissue and flap design [7, 8]. When the patient's single native breast volume exceeds this, then consideration is made for stacked PAP flaps. If bilateral reconstruction is being performed, and there is volume discrepancy, then consideration is then made for stacking the PAP flap with an abdominal flap (i.e. DIEP flap) to restore native breast volume.

3. Anatomy

As mentioned earlier, profunda artery perforators were well-described decades before the introduction into breast reconstruction, corroborated by cadaver dissection and imaging [4, 9–11]. The profunda artery branches from the common femoral artery several centimeters distal to the inguinal ligament. This source vessel runs in the posterior compartment and gives off on average three perforators that are within 7 cm from the inferior gluteal crease [4]. The most proximal perforator is often selected based on location and reliable perfusion. These perforators are invariably musculocutaneous, coursing through the adductor magnus muscle before irrigating the skin and subcutaneous tissues. The pedicle typically yields a pedicle length of 8–12 cm and caliber of 2.2 mm for artery and 2.7 mm for vein [8].

Regarding dimensions, Dr. Allen and his colleagues have reviewed their reconstructions and published in the largest clinical series using PAP flaps for breast reconstruction. The average flap weight was 367.4 g, and flap dimensions averaged 27.2 x 6.3 cm (**Figure 1**) [7].

4. Pre-operative imaging

Pre-operative imaging, via computed tomography angiography (CTA) or magnetic resonance angiography (MRA) is essential in elucidating perforator course and

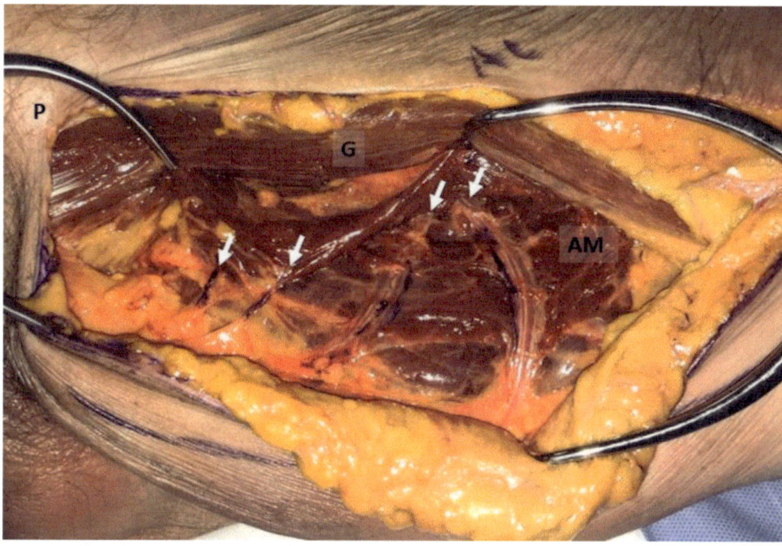

Figure 1.
Anatomic depiction of profunda artery perforators coursing through the adductor magnus muscle (P—pubis; G—gracilis; and M—adductor magnus).

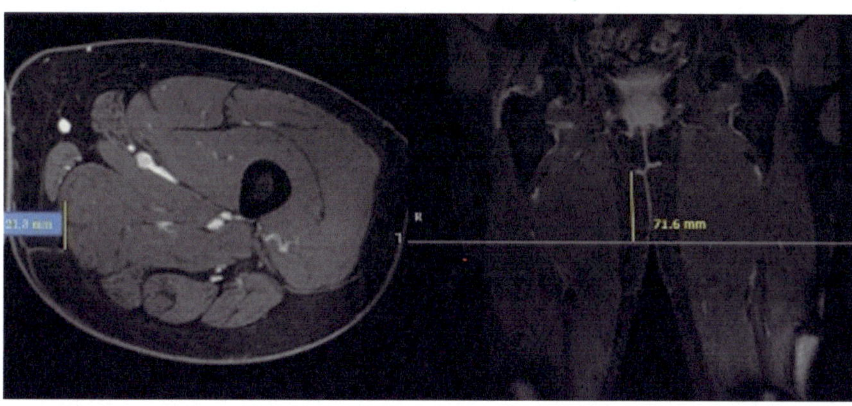

Figure 2.
MRA that displays distance from posterior border of gracilis to perforator at fascial exit on axial (left); distance from infra-gluteal gold to perforator at fascia exit on coronal (right). (Reprinted from [8]).

assisting with mapping the dissection and incisional planning. Confirmation of the desired perforator at the skin level is performed at the time of surgery with doppler ultrasound (**Figure 2**).

5. Standard profunda artery perforator flap markings and elevation

5.1 Transverse PAP flap

Since its introduction, approaching the PAP flap has been consistent. Variability does exist regarding orientation of the flap. The initial orientation was transverse in

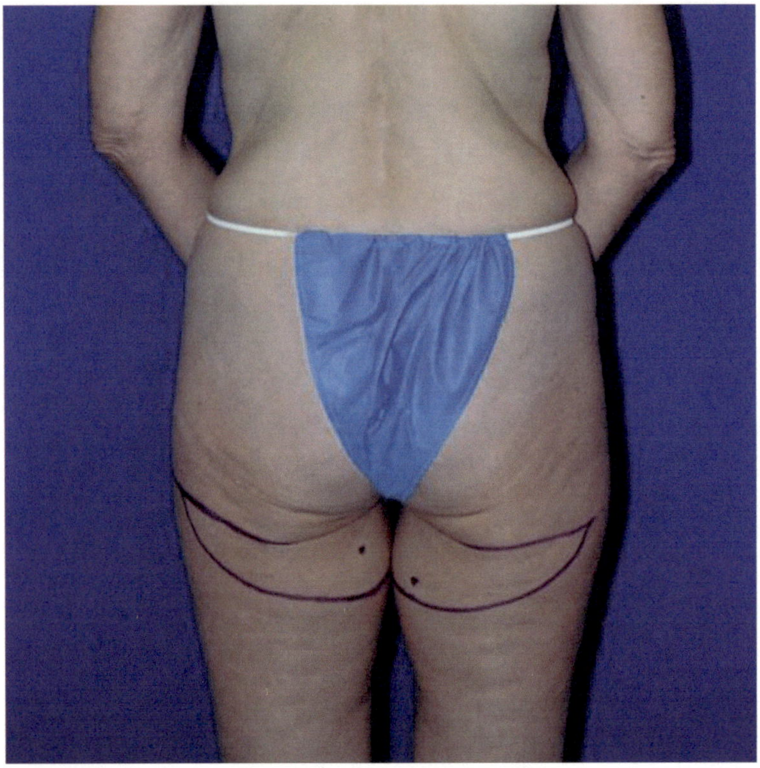

Figure 3.
Pre-operative picture with markings for transverse PAP flap showing the extend of posterior dissection. Perforators are marked on either side.

the upper thigh. This has been studied and expanded on, with alternative orientations including vertical, oblique, and combined vertical-transverse also known as the 'fleur-de-PAP' [12].

The standard transverse profunda artery perforator flap begins with marking the landmarks of the groin crease, mid-axial thigh, and inferior gluteal crease. Most commonly, the preferred perforator will be found within 7 cm of the inferior gluteal fold and within 4 cm of the posterior border of the gracilis. This is often identified with pre-operative imaging and confirmed with doppler ultrasound. Standard PAP flap markings are that of a transverse elliptical pattern performed with the patient standing. The width of the flap is determined by a pinch test (**Figure 3**).

5.2 Vertical PAP flap

The vertical design is oriented orthogonal to the transverse design. Anatomic landmarks include marking the pubic symphysis, the adductor longus and gracilis muscle borders. The perforator is marked using the doppler. The ellipse is centralized over the perforator and a pinch test is used to determine the width of the flap. This orientation is more commonly used by the senior author for multiple reasons—able to incorporate multiple perforators, assuring the dominant perforator is captured, lower chance for wound complications, less pain when sitting [8].

5.3 Flap elevation

Elevation of the flap begins with the anterior approach. The patient is positioned supine in lithotomy. The adductor longus and gracilis muscles are palpated and transposed to the skin surface. Dissection is carried down to the muscular fascia of the gracilis and proceeds posterior. In the anteromedial thigh the greater saphenous vein and tributaries will likely be encountered. Although these tributaries, if present, may aid venous drainage of the flap, supplemental outflow is typically not required and therefore they can be ligated with impunity. Once the gracilis muscle is identified, the dissection proceeds in the subfascial plane posteriorly. Skin perforators through the gracilis may be encountered and should be ligated. The septum between the gracilis and adductor magnus is important. The gracilis muscle is retracted anterior, and the adductor magnus fascia is incised and elevated. Dissection proceeds cautiously in the subfascial plane until the perforators are identified. Meticulous intramuscular dissection is performed to isolate the perforator(s) to the source vessel of the profunda artery and vein. This typically yields a pedicle length of 8–12 cm and caliber of 2.2 mm for artery and 2.7 mm for vein [4].

After circumferential dissection is completed, the anterior incision is stapled closed, and the posterior incision is completed. Care is taken not to bevel proximally as to preserve the ischial fat pad. The flap is harvested, weighed, and transplanted to the chest for microsurgical anastomosis. Most commonly, flap coning is performed prior to inset, and the flap may be completed de-epithelialized and buried in nipple-sparing mastectomies, or a skin paddle may be retained for monitoring and/or resurfacing of the breast skin (**Figure 4**).

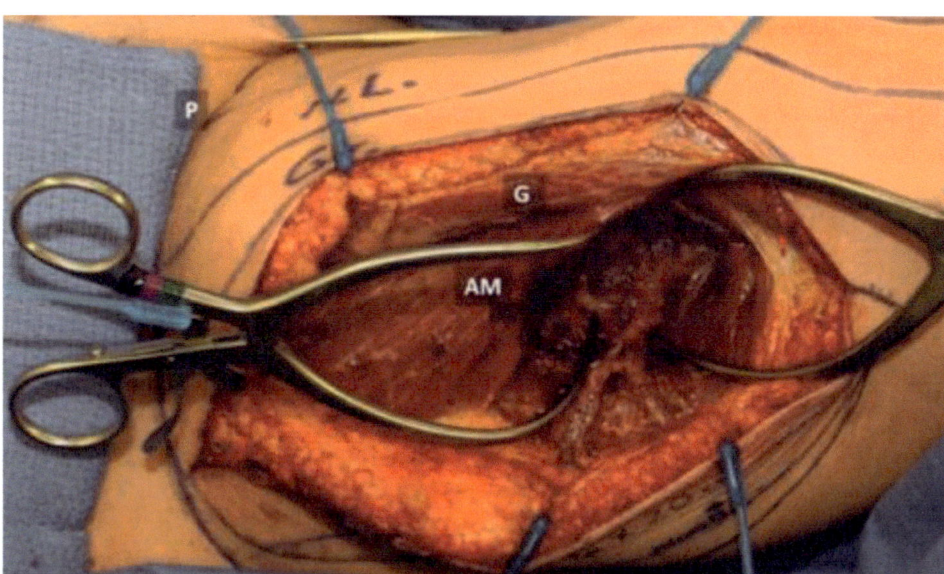

Figure 4.
Intraoperative dissection of the left vertical PAP flap. Perforators can be seen piercing the adductor magnus (AM). Flap characteristics: : 367 g; Average flap dimensions: 27 × 6 cm; Average pedicle length: 10.2 cm; Average artery diameter: 2.2 mm; and Average vein diameter: 2.8 mm.

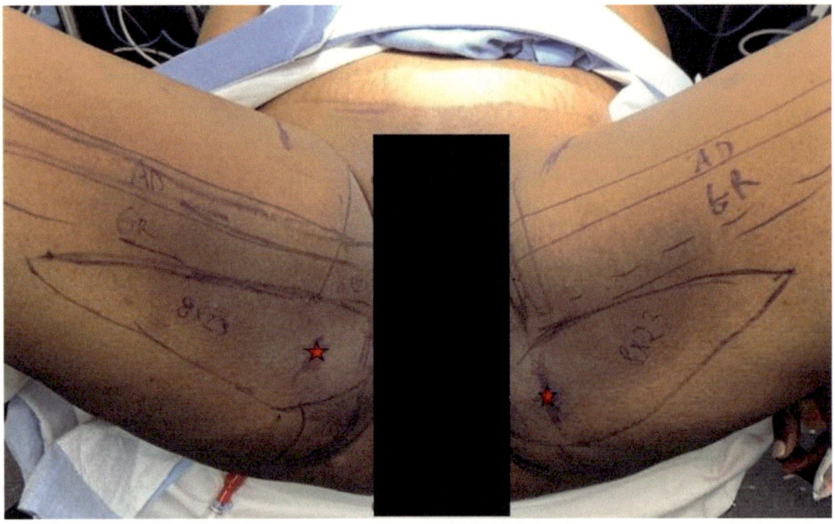

Figure 5.
Pre-operative picture of markings for an extended PAP or 'fleur-de-PAP' including both vertical and transverse extension centered over the perforators (stars).

5.4 Extended or 'Fleur-de-PAP' modification

The 'fleur-de-PAP' is a mosaic expanded modification of the standard PAP flap. Specifically, it includes both a transverse and vertical component to incorporate additional tissue [12, 13]. This increases volume at the cost of a longitudinal scar in the medial mid-axial thigh and a 'T'-junction closure. Markings are similar, and emphasis should be placed on location of the dominant perforator to establish a central point for which the transverse and vertical components converge. Width is also determined by a skin pinch. Flap elevation is identical to that of the standard profunda artery perforator flap harvest (**Figure 5**).

6. Flap contouring

The goal of breast reconstruction is to emulate natural esthetics. Achieving this not only requires technical finesse in microsurgery, but esthetic prowess. This often requires multiple stages of surgery, however as reconstructive surgeons become more proficient in the operating room, less time is spent on microsurgery and more time can be dedicated to contouring the breast mound at the first stage. This is evident in outcomes seen with PAP flaps. The elliptical orientation of the flaps lends itself to being molded immediately, regardless of the need for skin paddle. The fat is more supple and yields to contouring. This is often achieved on the back table prior to inset. If the patient is fortunate to have a nipple sparing mastectomy, the entire flap is de-epithelialized and folded to produce an esthetically pleasing breast mound. Otherwise, a skin paddle is left to monitor the flap. The three-dimensional construct is maintained with absorbable internal sutures and does not require the addition of supplemental materials such as meshes or slings (**Figure 6**).

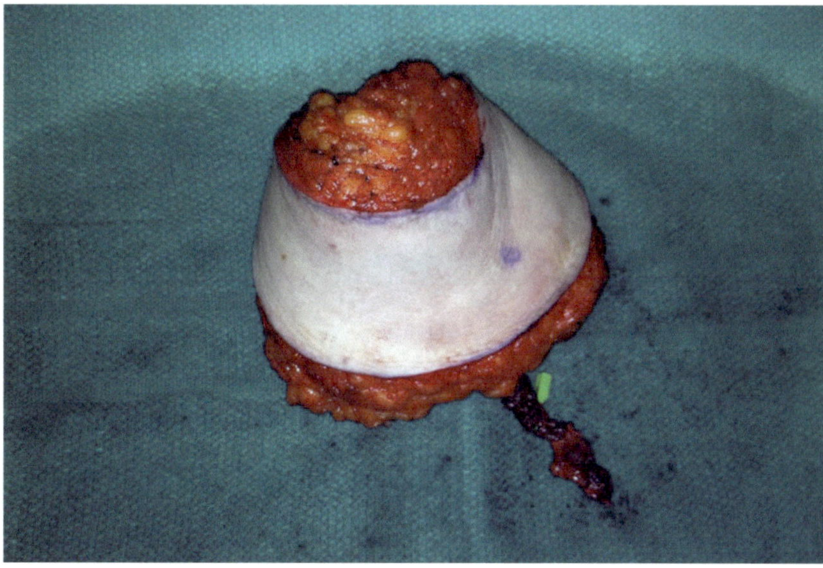

Figure 6.
Intra-operative contouring of a single PAP flap into an esthetic breast mound.

7. Stacking flaps

Modern advancements in microsurgery have provided ample options for breast reconstruction, such that flap design can be personalized for each patient based on anatomy of both the breasts and donor sites. Trends over the last decade at our institution have shown an increase in stacked flap reconstructions. There are several variables to consider when approaching stacked flaps: (1) breast volume, (2) unilateral versus bilateral, (3) donor site availability, (4) donor site volume. An algorithmic approach can assist the pre-operative decision-making process [14, 15].

The most common scenario for performing stacked PAP flaps is either: restoration of volume in a unilateral breast reconstruction (PAP + PAP) or need for additional volume to augment bilateral breast reconstruction (DIEP + PAP).

The preferred orientation for stacking PAP flaps in a unilateral breast reconstruction is to perform the first anastomosis between the ipsilateral PAP flap and antegrade internal mammary vessels, followed by the contralateral PAP flap to the retrograde internal mammary vessels. It is important to note that contouring the flap on a sterile flap table should be done prior to the microsurgical anastomosis to facilitate ease of inset afterwards (**Figure 7**).

There are multiple options for microsurgical anastomosis when combining the PAP and DIEP flap [16]. The bulk of the flap volume will come from the DIEP flap, which is centralized on the breast. If the volume between the DIEP flap and the PAP flap are similar, they can be combined to form a mound with internal sutures, and oriented such that the pedicle of the DIEP flap can lie in line with the antegrade internal mammary vessels, and the PAP flap pedicle lie in line with the retrograde vessels. Alternatively, if the DIEP flap is significantly large, it is used to reconstruct most of the central breast and upper pole, while the PAP flap augments the inferior pole volume (**Figure 8**).

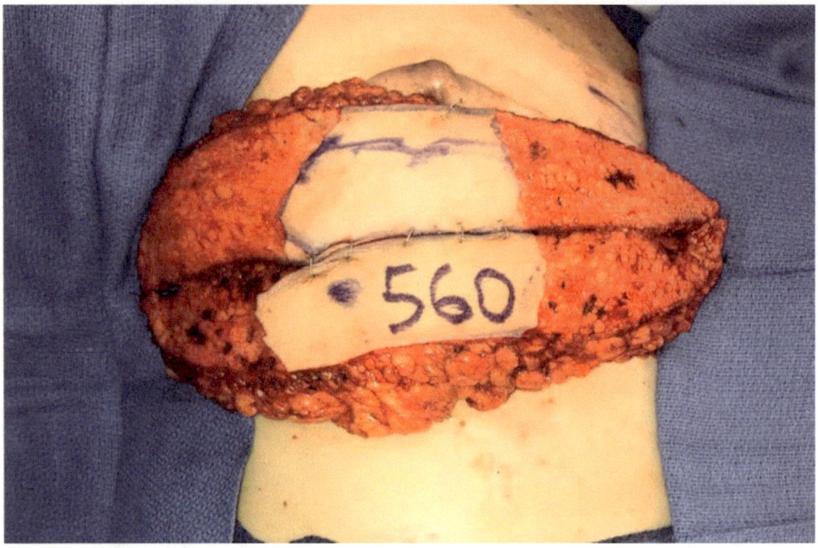

Figure 7.
Intraoperative picture of stacked PAP flaps with combined weight of 560 g.

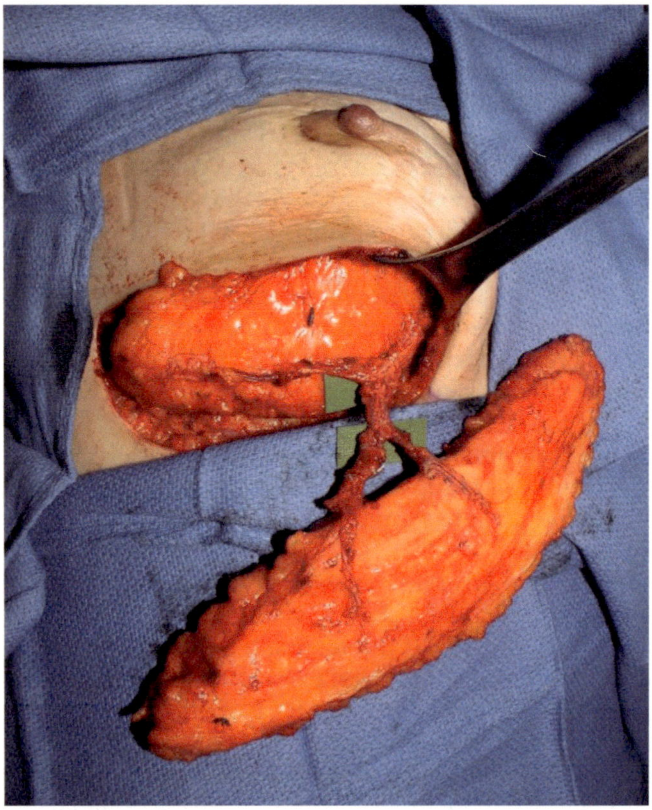

Figure 8.
Intraoperative picture of stacked DIEP and PAP flap. The green microgrids are placed under the PAP pedicle. The DIEP flap has been de-epithelialized and inset, and the PAP flap restores the lower pole volume.

7.1 Tips and tricks

- Pre-operative imaging (CTA/MRA) is critical for perforator mapping and surgical efficiency.
- Limit flap width (~7 cm) to avoid tight incisional closure and wound healing issues.
- Identify posterior border and reflect the gracilis anteriorly, then enter the subfascial plane of the adductor magnus to identify perforators.
- Avoid beveling superiorly to retain the ischial fat pad and avoid sitting discomfort.
- For single flap reconstruction, use intra-flap absorbable sutures to create an esthetic breast mound prior to inset.
- For stacked reconstruction, align the flaps flat and side by side to gain additional base width.
- Consider two flaps for single breast reconstruction at primary procedure.

8. Donor site management

The profunda artery perforator flap harvests no muscle and therefore has minimal donor site morbidity. However, the location is in a dynamic area of the lower extremity and is prone to tensional forces and edema. For these reasons, the donor site needs to be managed appropriately. Limited undermining of skin flaps helps facilitate a tension-free closure while preventing seroma formation. A closed suction drain is always used. Quilting sutures are beneficial and involves suturing the superficial fascia to the deep fascia. Compression garments or ACE wraps are used.

9. Complications

Flap-related complications are low regarding breast reconstruction with PAP flaps. Profunda artery perforator perfusion is robust and therefore the risk of fat necrosis generally is minimal, both in incidence and volume. Fat necrosis is mostly seen at the tips of the flap and can be avoided by careful intra-operative clinical assessment and prophylactic excisional debridement of presumptive nonviable fat.

Donor site complications are more common. These include, but are not limited to, seroma, delayed wound healing, dehiscence, prolonged edema, dysesthesia, adverse scarring [5, 7].

Seroma should be distinguished easily from prolonged edema, which may also occur. This is done with a clinical exam and confirmed with ultrasound imaging. Prevention is the primary focus. This includes limiting undermining, closed suction drain, quilting sutures, layered closure, and post-operative compression garments. Persistent or recurrent seromas are treated with aspiration and/or drain placement as needed.

Due to the dynamic nature of the surgical site with ambulation, as well as being located near an intertriginous zone, delayed wound healing can occur. Dehiscence is much less common. Appropriate pre-operative planning with pinch-test and conservative skin markings support tension-free closure and routine wound healing. The Fleur-de-PAP is more susceptible to wound healing complications due to the creation of a T-junction with the skin flaps.

Prolonged edema is typically caused by disruption of major lymphatic channels in the lower extremity. The PAP flap dissection avoids the femoral triangle and major lymphatic channels; therefore, the risk is quite low. Preserving the greater saphenous vein, tributaries, and surrounding lymphatics can help prevent edema. Early ambulation with compression dressings or garments is standard of care.

Post-surgical dysesthesia, like the infraumbilical skin after DIEP flap, is a result of cutaneous nerve disruption after flap elevation and is best treated with reassurance and time.

Adverse scarring, namely widened or hypertrophic scars, can occur and is thought to be due to motion and dynamic tension at the suture line, like a thigh lift or brachioplasty.

10. Discussion

Since its introduction to breast reconstruction in 2010, the profunda artery perforator flap has been a reliable autologous alternative to the DIEP flap within the armamentarium of the reconstructive microsurgeon. It has also been an important additional method when the DIEP flap is not enough. The PAP boasts a large skin paddle (average 27 x 6 cm), ample pedicle length and good caliber, and mild-to-moderate volume of soft, pliable tissue. The ability to harvest the flap from a supine position with a two-team approach increases efficiency. The vascular anatomy is constant which has been corroborated with the routine use of pre-operative CT/MR angiography. The donor site results in acceptable scars with minimal exposure and complication rate. This is expounded by the recently described 'fleur-de-PAP' which enhances the volume at the cost of minimal excess scarring. Pedicle length and caliber enhances its utility in stacked flap procedures. The ability to immediately mold the flap into an esthetically excellent three-dimensional breast mound cannot be overstated.

The primary disadvantage of the flap is volume. However, this can be circumvented with proper patient selection and flap planning, including stacked flaps, hybrid procedures, and subsequent fat grafting (**Figure 9A–D**).

11. Conclusion

The profunda artery perforator flap is an alternative approach to flap-based breast reconstruction. As breast reconstruction continues to advance, the prevalence of alternative approaches such as the PAP flap will increase. Familiarity with anatomy, microsurgical elevation, contouring and donor site management is critical to achieving excellent esthetic outcomes and professional success.

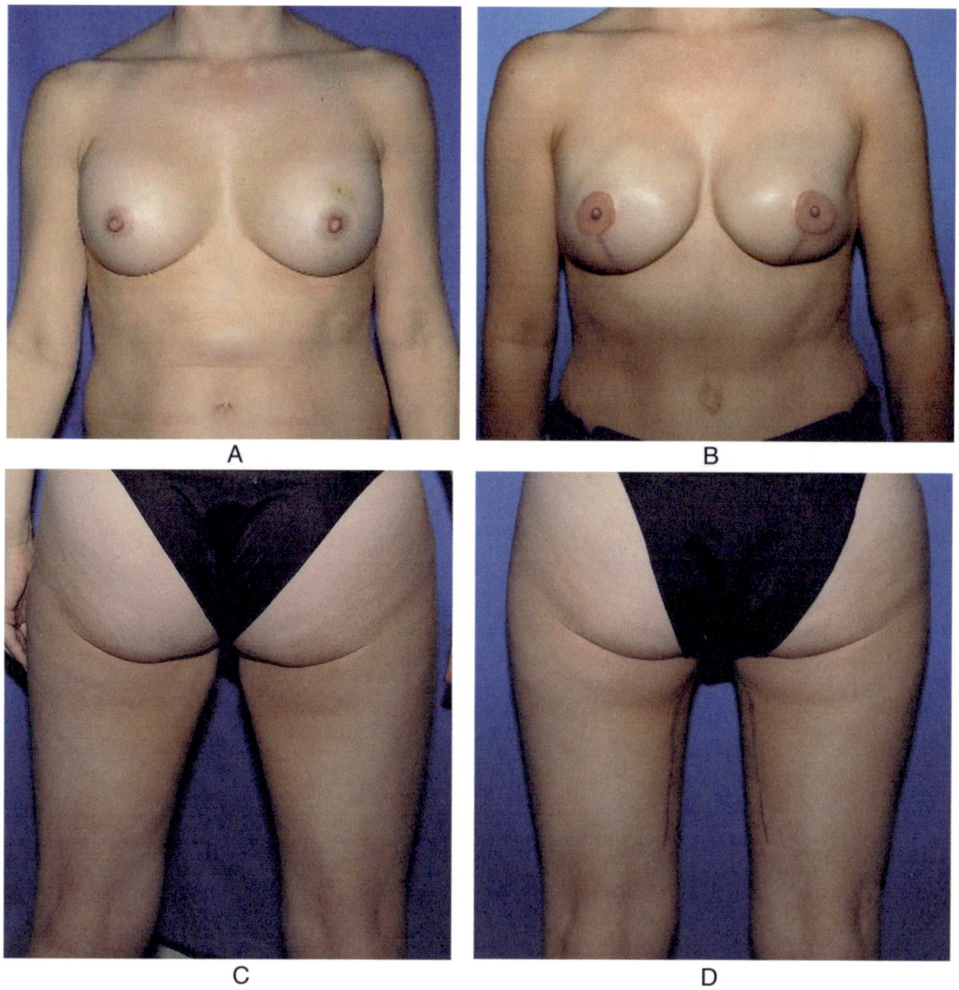

Figure 9.
(A, B) Pre and post-operative images of a patient with left breast cancer who underwent stacked DIEP and PAP flap reconstruction of the bilateral breasts. (C and D) Pre and post-operative images well-hidden PAP flap donor sites, without disruption of the infragluteal fold. (Reprinted from Artz et al. [8]).

Acknowledgements

We would like to acknowledge Dr. Robert Allen for his incredible contributions to both this chapter and the innovation of the profunda artery perforator flap in breast reconstruction. We would also like to acknowledge his home institution, Louisiana State University Division of Plastic Surgery for their supportive efforts, and where Dr. Allen continues to contribute to the field of reconstructive microsurgery.

Conflict of interest

The authors declare no conflicts of interest.

Appendices and nomenclature

PAP	profunda artery perforator
DIEP	deep inferior epigastric artery perforator
CTA	computed tomography angiography
MRA	magnetic resonance angiography

Author details

Michael Borrero, Robert Allen and Hugo St. Hilaire*
Louisiana State University Health Sciences, New Orleans, LA, USA

*Address all correspondence to: hsthil@lsuhsc.edu

IntechOpen

© 2023 The Author(s). Licensee IntechOpen. This chapter is distributed under the terms of the Creative Commons Attribution License (http://creativecommons.org/licenses/by/3.0), which permits unrestricted use, distribution, and reproduction in any medium, provided the original work is properly cited.

References

[1] Hurwitz DJ, Swartz WM, Mathes SJ. The gluteal thigh flap: A reliable, sensate flap for the closure of buttock and perineal wounds. Plastic and Reconstructive Surgery. 1981;**68**:521-532

[2] Song YG, Chen GZ, Song YL. The free thigh flap: A new free flap concept based on the septocutaneous artery. British Journal of Plastic Surgery. 1984;**37**:149-159

[3] Angrigiani C, Grilli D, Thorne CH. The adductor flap: A new method for transferring posterior and medial thigh skin. Plastic and Reconstructive Surgery. 2001;**107**:1725-1731

[4] Saad A, Sadeghi A, Allen RJ. The anatomic basis of the profunda femoris artery perforator flap: A new option for autologous breast reconstruction—A cadaveric and computer tomography angiogram study. Journal of Reconstructive Microsurgery. 2012;**28**:381-386

[5] Allen RJ, Haddock NT, Ahn CY, et al. Breast reconstruction with the profunda artery perforator flap. Plastic and Reconstructive Surgery. 2012;**129**:16e-23e

[6] Massey MF, Spiegel AJ, Levine JL, et al. Perforator flaps: Recent experience, current trends, and future directions based on 3974 microsurgical breast reconstructions. Plastic and Reconstructive Surgery. 2009;**124**:737-751

[7] Allen RJ, Lee ZH, Mayo JL, et al. The profunda artery perforator flap experience for breast reconstruction. Plastic and Reconstructive Surgery. 2016;**138**:968-975

[8] Artz JD, Atamian EK, Mulloy C, et al. Use of the vertical profunda artery perforator flap to capture the dominant perforator: A cadaver dissection and imaging study. Journal of Reconstructive Microsurgery. 2022;**38**(4):284-291. DOI: 10.1055/s-0041-1731764

[9] Haddock NT, Greaney P, Otterburn D, et al. Predicting perforator location on preoperative imaging for the profunda artery perforator flap. Microsurgery. 2012;**32**:507-511

[10] DeLong MR, Hughes DB, Bond JE, et al. A detailed evaluation of the anatomical variations of the profunda artery perforator flap using computed tomographic angiograms. Plastic and Reconstructive Surgery. 2014;**134**:186e-192e

[11] Ahmadzadeh R, Bergeron L, Tang M, et al. The posterior thigh perforator flap or profunda femoris artery perforator flap. Plastic and Reconstructive Surgery. 2007;**119**:194-200, discussion 201-202

[12] Bourn L, Torabi R, Stalder MW, et al. Mosaic Fleur-de-profunda artery perforator flap for autologous breast reconstruction. Plastic and Reconstructive Surgery. Global Open. 2019;**7**(03):e2166

[13] Dayan JH, Allen RJ Jr. Neurotized diagonal profunda artery perforator flaps for breast reconstruction. Plastic and Reconstructive Surgery. Global Open. 2019;**7**:e2463

[14] Mayo JL, Canizares O, Torabi R, et al. Expanding the applications of the profunda artery perforator flap. Plastic and Reconstructive Surgery. 2016;**137**:663-669

[15] Levine JL, Soueid NE, Allen RJ. Algorithm for autologous breast

reconstruction for partial mastectomy defects. Plastic and Reconstructive Surgery. 2005;**116**:762-767

[16] Mayo JL, Allen RJ, Sadeghi A. Four-flap breast reconstruction: Bilateral stacked DIEP and PAP flaps. Plastic and Reconstructive Surgery. Global Open. 2015;**3**:e383

Chapter 9

Application of CT Angiography in Delayed DIEP Flap Breast Reconstruction

Xu Yuanbing, Pan Dai and Xu Hua

Abstract

How to safely and effectively locate, select and dissect the perforator vessels is the biggest difficulty in the preparation of DIEP flap. Preoperative CTA was used to evaluate the perforators of the DIEP flap. The CTA data were imported into the image analysis software to select the dominant perforators of the flap before operation, and to determine the anatomical information such as the diameter of the perforator vessel, the course of the perforator in the muscle, and the location of the perforator exit point, so as to guide the operation. In summary, CTA technology can accurately provide detailed anatomical information of perforator vessels, facilitate surgical design, reduce intraoperative perforator selection and dissection time, reduce the risk of secondary surgical exploration, and have a high imaging and surgical consistency rate, especially for patients with a history of abdominal surgery, CTA is of higher value. Therefore, CTA examination is worthy of clinical application in delayed DIEP breast flap reconstruction.

Keywords: computed tomographic angiography, deep inferior epigastric perforator, breast reconstruction, delayed, breast cancer

1. Introduction

Breast reconstruction is becoming more popular under the basis of tumor safety. The rate of immediate or delayed reconstruction following breast cancer surgery has grown dramatically [1, 2]. Deep inferior epigastric perforator (DIEP) flap has become the gold standard in autologous breast reconstruction due to low donor site problems and significant abdominal esthetic improvement [3]. While DIEP flap surgery has become commonplace, the anatomy of the deep inferior epigastric artery perforator is very diverse, and flap perforator selection remains difficult. Color Doppler ultrasonography was the first approach used to evaluate perforators in DIEP [4]. Nevertheless, due to its strong subjectivity, time-consuming nature, high false positive rate of preoperative perforator evaluation, and lack of local anatomical features, its applicability is limited to some extent. Till date, computed tomography angiography (CTA) has been an essential assessment approach prior to DIEP surgery [5, 6]. CTA can provide more detailed preoperative anatomical information than color Doppler ultrasound examination, which can help to

IntechOpen

better select the dominant perforator of the flap before surgery, clarify the diameter of the perforator vessels, the characteristics of the perforator vessels in the muscle, and the location of the perforator point, so as to effectively guide the operation process [7].

2. Research method

2.1 Grouping overview

This study has collected clinical data from 298 female patients undergoing breast reconstruction surgery following breast cancer surgery, ranging in age from 25 to 67 years (mean age 42.2 ± 8.28 years). Before undergoing reconstructive surgery, all patients had conventional tumor therapy and were in a stable disease phase. In January 2016 and January 2018, 92 patients (US group) had their data gathered. Prior to surgery, these patients were subjected to a color Doppler ultrasound examination to examine abdominal vascular perforators using a GE Logiq 700 ultrasonography machine with a probe frequency of 10–13 MHz and a color Doppler frequency of 7.5 MHz, with a maximum velocity of 2 cm/s. The focus of the examination was to accurately detect where the target perforator vessels exited the deep fascia and entered the subcutaneous fat layer, and then to label the matching surface projection. As the observation group, data from 206 patients was gathered between January 2018 and January 2021 (CTA group). These patients underwent abdominal vascular perforator evaluation prior to surgery using a Philips Brilliance 256i CT scanner, which used a non-ionic iodine contrast agent (iopromide) with a volume of 90–100 mL and an injection rate of 4 mL/s, introduced via a vein on the back of the hand or at the elbow. The following CTA settings were employed with a single high-pressure injector: 120 kVp, 250 mA, detector 128 × 0.625 mm, pitch 0.977, 512 × 512 matrix, and a 350 mm field of view.

2.2 CTA image data processing

The HOROS software was used to evaluate the data and establish the location and trajectory of perforator vessels, which were then marked on the patient's body surface.

2.3 Research indexs

Baseline data were collected for both groups and compared, including age, body mass index (BMI), history of hypertension or diabetes, history of tumor chemotherapy, chest wall radiation history, abdominal surgery history, smoking history, and single/double pedicle flap blood supply. In addition, intraoperative and postoperative evaluation indices were statistically analyzed. Intraoperative evaluation indices included the number of perforators located preoperatively, the number of perforators utilized during the surgery, the decision-making time for perforators, perforator dissection time, flap harvesting time, flap total weight, and total operation time. The postoperative evaluation indices included abdominal incision infection rate, fat necrosis rate, re-exploration rate, and complete flap necrosis rate.

3. Surgical procedure

3.1 Preoperative localization of DIEP flap perforator

Patients in the US group had US examinations the day before the surgery, with the US group getting surface markings of perforator arteries directly under color doppler ultrasound guidance. CT vascular imaging examinations were done in the CT room for the CTA group, and the physician duplicated the DICOM files and loaded them into the HOROS program on their mobile phone or a personal computer. The imaging processing system was used to determine the dominant perforator, and the position of the chosen dominant perforator was written on the body surface centered on the level of the umbilicus.

3.2 Preoperative scribing

Based on the shape of the patient's contralateral breast, the reconstruction of the breast fold and the separation area of the inner and outer sides of the affected breast were marked on the body surface prior to surgery.

3.3 Receiving area pretreatment

During surgery, the patient was positioned supine, and the scar tissue on the chest wall was addressed, as well as the cavity of the breast flap divided. The third rib cartilage was regularly resected to reveal the recipient vessels within the chest wall.

3.4 Preparation of the donor site

A DIEP flap was harvested and dissected after a perforator site close to the marked area was identified. The power of the electric scalpel was lowered to measure and mark the target perforator vessel again with the center at the level of the umbilicus on the anterior sheath surface. The perforator vessel was carefully dissected and separated, and the DIEP flap was obtained. The upper and lower abdominal wall tissues were freed, the abdominal wall was reshaped, the umbilical hernia was reconstructed, and the abdominal incision was closed.

3.5 Microvascular anastomosis and breast reconstruction

The recipient artery and vein were dissected and reserved, with the distal ends being ligated and the proximal ends being clamped. The blood vessels within the chest wall were trimmed. The flap was moved to the breast defect site and temporarily fixed, and the veins and arteries below the abdominal wall were trimmed. Microscopic vascular anastomosis was performed using 9-0 or 10-0 prolene suture thread. The patency of the anastomosis was checked. After the flap blood supply was established, the shape of the breast was formed.

4. Research results

4.1 Comparison of preoperative baseline data between the two groups

Among 298 patients undergoing delayed DIEP flap breast reconstruction, the overall survival rate of the flap was 99.33% (296/298). There were no significant differences between the two groups in age, BMI, history of underlying diseases, history of tumor chemotherapy, history of chest wall radiotherapy, history of abdominal surgery, history of smoking, and blood supply of the flap (uni/bi-pedicle) ($P > 0.05$) (**Table 1**).

4.2 Comparison of intraoperative and postoperative outcome indexes between the two groups

In the observation group, the number of preoperative location perforations was (2.90 ± 1.13), while that in the control group was (3.21 ± 1.46), and the difference was statistically significant. In terms of perforator decision time and perforator anatomy time, the observation group was shorter than the control group ($P < 0.001$), as shown in **Table 2**. The acquisition time of donor flap was (50.05 ± 10.94) min in the observation group and (84.8 ± 15.44) min in the control group. Donor site flap

Factors	CTA group	US group	F/χ^2	*P* value
Age/year	41.78 ± 9.06	40.94 ± 8.61	1.25	0.27
BMI	24.34 ± 3.20	24.21 ± 2.86	0.71	0.40
Basic disease			0.098	0.754
With	25	10		
Without	181	82		
Chemotherapy			0.281	0.596
With	168	69		
Without	48	23		
Chest wall radiotherapy			0.001	0.977
With	72	32		
Without	134	60		
Abdominal surgery			0.264	0.608
With	82	36		
Without	124	56		
Smoking			0.017	0.895
Yes	4	2		
No	202	90		
Blood supply of flap			0.128	0.720
Unipedicle	85	40		
Bipedicle	121	52		

Table 1.
Comparison of baseline data between two groups.

DOI: http://dx.doi.org/10.5772/intechopen.112913

Indicators	CTA group	US group	F/χ^2	*P* value
Number of preoperative location perforations	2.90 ± 1.13	3.21 ± 1.46	6.46	0.012
Number of intraoperative choice perforations	2.26 ± 0.92	2.49 ± 0.96	0.907	0.342
Perforation choice time (min)	9.14 ± 3.38	26.73 ± 6.54	49.42	<0.001
Perforation anatomy time (min)	40.92 ± 9.98	58.11 ± 14.44	19.64	<0.001
Donor site flap acquisition time (min)	50.05 ± 10.94	84.8 ± 15.44	15.56	<0.001
Flap weight (g)	730.62 ± 127.31	718.25 ± 129.36	0.005	0.942
Total operation time (min)	294.20 ± 68.51	328.74 ± 68.69	0.058	0.809
Abdominal incision infection			0.199	0.656
Yes	3	2		
No	203	90		
Fat necrosis			0.404	0.525
Yes	6	4		
No	200	88		
Secondary surgical exploration			11.501	<0.001
Yes	6	12		
No	200	80		
Complete flap necrosis				
Yes	0	2		0.095
No	206	90		

Table 2.
Comparison of intraoperative and postoperative indicators between two groups.

acquisition time was shorter in the observation group, and the difference was statistically significant ($P < 0.001$). There was no significant difference in the total operation time between the two groups ($P = 0.809$) (**Figure 1**). The total weight of the flap was (730.62 ± 127.31) g in the observation group and (718.25 ± 129.36) g in the control group, showing no difference.

In the comparison of postoperative complications between the two groups, there were no statistical differences in abdominal incision infection rate, fat necrosis rate and flap complete necrosis rate ($P > 0.05$). In the comparison of secondary surgical exploration rate, the CTA group was lower than the US group ($P < 0.001$) (**Figure 2**).

4.3 Patients in the two groups were stratified according to whether there was a history of abdominal surgery

Stratified comparisons were made with or without a history of abdominal surgery. The experimental data were divided into four groups: ① CTA + NAS (non-abdominal surgery); ② CTA + AS; ③ US + NAS; ④ US + AS. The results showed that the time and total operation time of the flap were increased in both the CTA group and the US group in patients with a history of abdominal surgery ($P < 0.05$). For patients with a

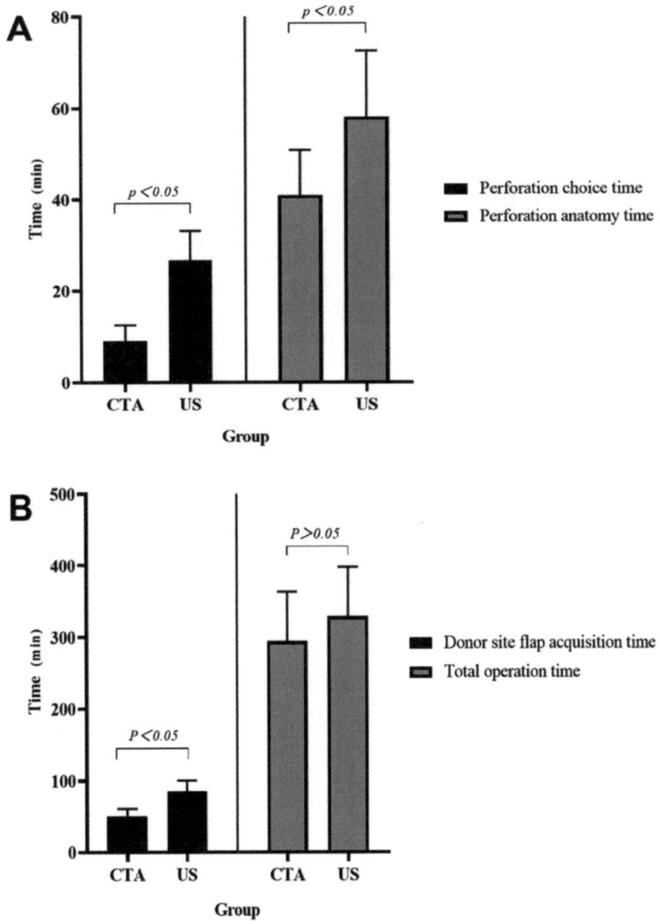

Figure 1.
Comparison of key intraoperative indicators.

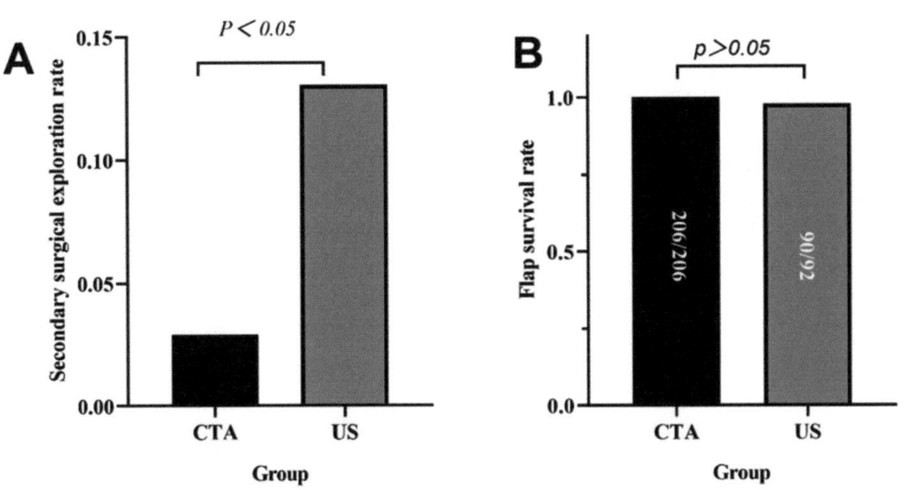

Figure 2.
Comparison of key postoperative indicators.

history of abdominal surgery, the time and total operation time of the flap in the CTA group were lower than those in the US group ($P < 0.05$). For patients with no history of abdominal surgery, the time of flap resection in CTA group was lower than that in US group ($P < 0.05$), and there was no significant difference in total operation time ($P > 0.05$) (**Table 3**).

4.4 Analysis of consistency rate of imaging surgery

Among 206 flaps in the observation group, the perforator selection in 200 flaps was related to CTA, and the consistency rate of imaging operation was 97.09%; among 92 flaps in the control group, the perforator selection in 40 flaps was related to US, and the consistency rate of imaging operation was 43.48%, with statistical significance ($P < 0.001$) (**Table 4**).

4.5 Typical cases

The female patient, 65 years old, was admitted to hospital due to "left breast defect 10 years after left breast cancer surgery." Specialized physical examination on admission showed: chest: postoperative changes of left breast cancer, absence of left breast, surgical scar about 15.0×1.0 cm in length visible on left chest wall, good healing, no skin ulceration, nodules and other abnormalities. There was mild drooping of the right breast, no obvious abnormal nodules in it, no obvious enlarged lymph nodes in the bilateral axilla and the upper and lower clavicular region. Abdomen: The patient's abdomen was slightly elevated, and the longitudinal surgical scar about 10.0*1.0 cm in length was visible in the lower abdomen. Preoperative images are shown in **Figure 3A**. After admission, the general condition assessment was completed, and no obvious contraindications were found, so the left breast reconstruction with DIEP flap was performed under general anesthesia. Before surgery, the patients underwent CTA

Groups	Perforation anatomy time(min)	*P* value	Total operation time(min)	*P* value
① CTA + NAS	32.06 ± 7.96	0.023[a]	288.46 ± 58.34	0.040[e]
② CTA + AS	42.36 ± 10.06	<0.001[b]	300.06 ± 60.29	0.018[f]
③ US + NAS	50.98 ± 13.02	<0.001[c]	304.78 ± 64.58	0.248[g]
④ US + AS	68.30 ± 15.08	0.012[d]	332.03 ± 70.28	0.014[h]

Note: Comparison of perforation anatomy time between different groups: a is ①vs②comparison; b is ③vs④ comparison; c is ①vs③ comparison; d is ②vs④ comparison. Total operation time (min): e is ①vs②comparison; f is ③vs④ comparison; g is ①vs③ comparison; and h is ②vs④ comparison.

Table 3.
Stratification analysis according to the history of abdominal surgery between two groups.

Groups	Total number of cases	Conformed cases	Accordance rate (%)	*P* value
US	92	40	43.48	<0.001
CTA	206	200	97.09	

Table 4.
Comparison of the consistency rate of imaging surgery between two groups.

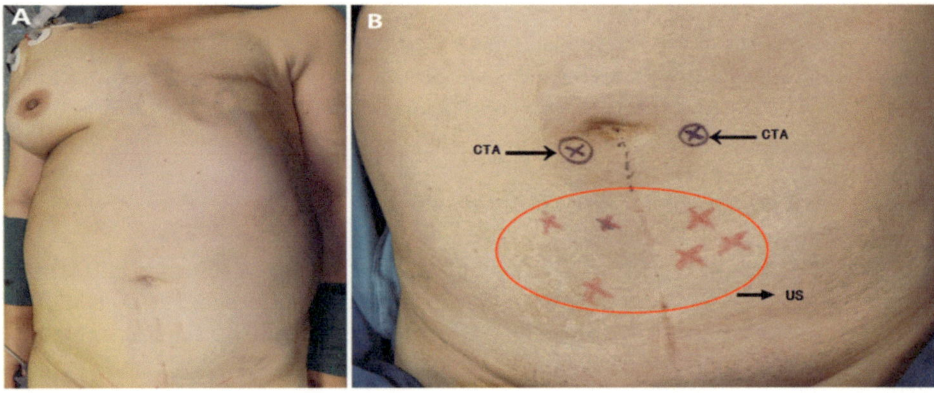

Figure 3.
Preoperative thoracic and abdominal images of the patient. (A) Preoperative image, and (B) In the preoperative positioning image, the black arrow shows the vessel perforator located by CTA, and the red mark in the red circle is the vessel perforator location point evaluated by preoperative ultrasound.

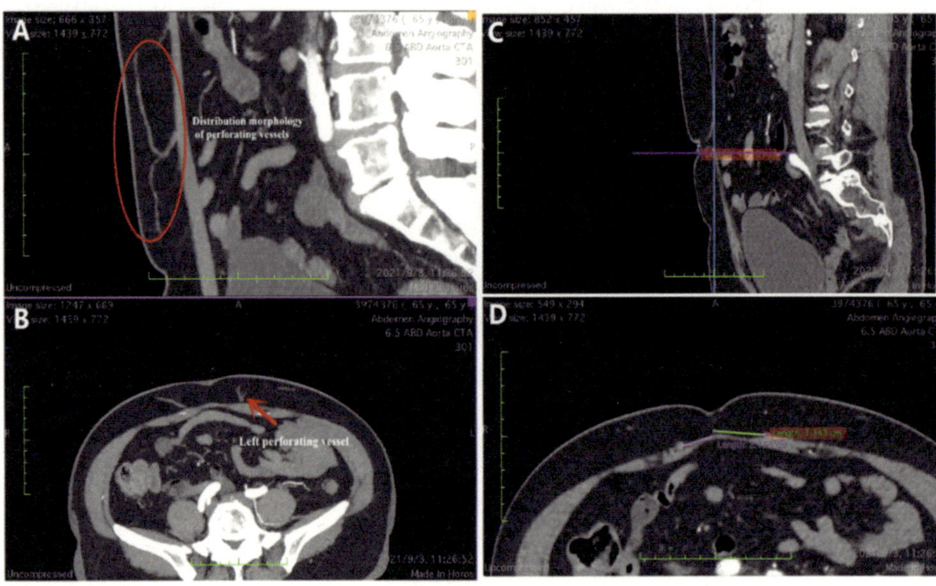

Figure 4.
CTA images of perforator vessels. (A) The left perforator was in the shape direction of the flap, (B) The exit point of the left perforator flap, (C) Vertical distance between sagittal perforating branches and the center of the umbilicus, and (D) Vertical distance between left and right perforating branches and the center of the umbilicus.

examination first, and then abdominal ultrasound examination. The body surface identification of the dominant perforator was performed in the blind state, respectively, as shown in **Figure 3B**. Before surgery, the location of the dominant perforator on the left and right sides was calculated in horizontal, coronal and sagittal positions with the umbilical level as the center, respectively, as shown in **Figure 4**. During the operation, CTA navigation technology was combined to accurately locate the corresponding perforator vessels, as shown in **Figure 5**. The perforator vessels of both sides of the flap and DIEP flap were completely free for flap shaping and breast shaping, as shown in

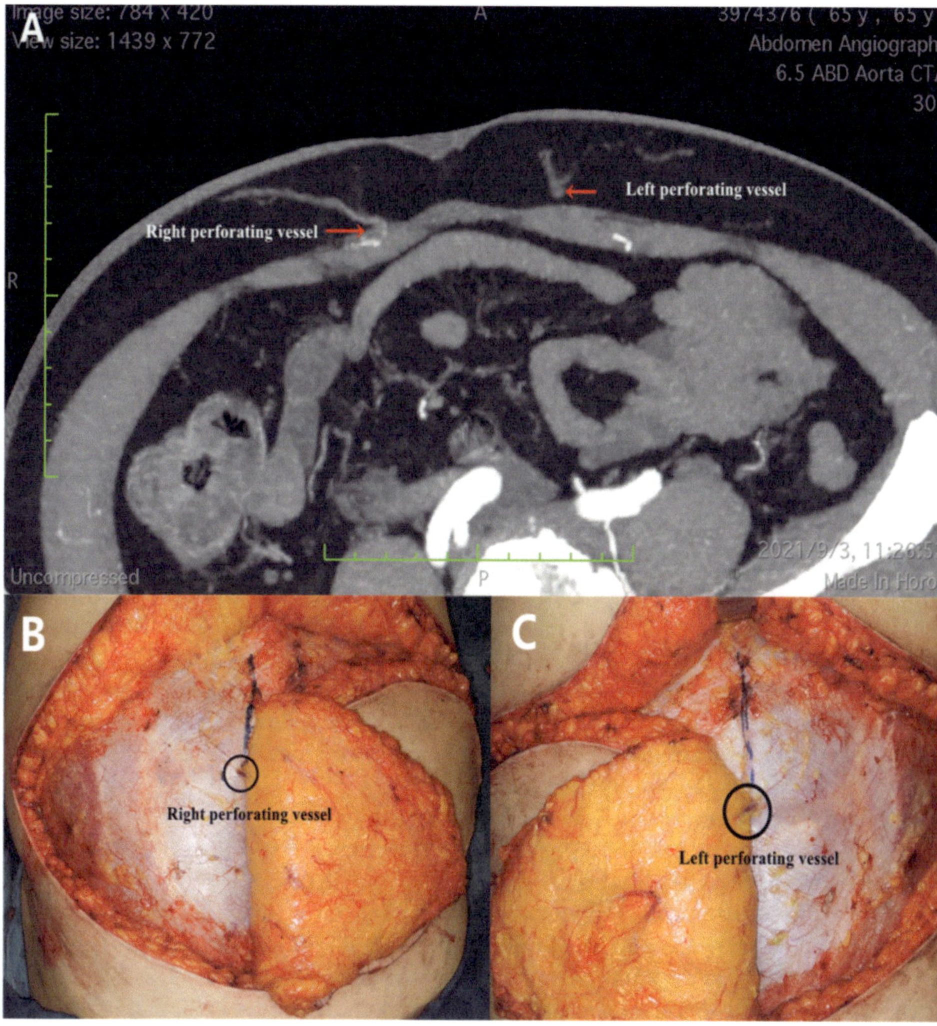

Figure 5.
Perforator vessel image-real comparison. (A) The red arrow shows the left and right perforations respectively, and (B and C) The actual right and left perforations calculated according to CTA during the operation respectively.

Figure 6. The surgery was successful. The chest drainage tube was removed 3 days after surgery, and the abdominal drainage tube was removed 5 days after surgery.

5. Discussion

The DIEP flap has numerous benefits in breast restoration, including big tissue acquisition, tissue similarity in the donor region, full preservation of rectus abdominis and anterior sheath tissue, and so on. It can also help with abdominal wall reconstruction in individuals who have abdominal fat accumulation. DIEP is currently the favored flap for autologous tissue breast surgery. However, due to its technological complexity, lengthy operation time, convoluted intraoperative links, and high postoperative complications, the operation of the DIEP flap is limited to some degree [8].

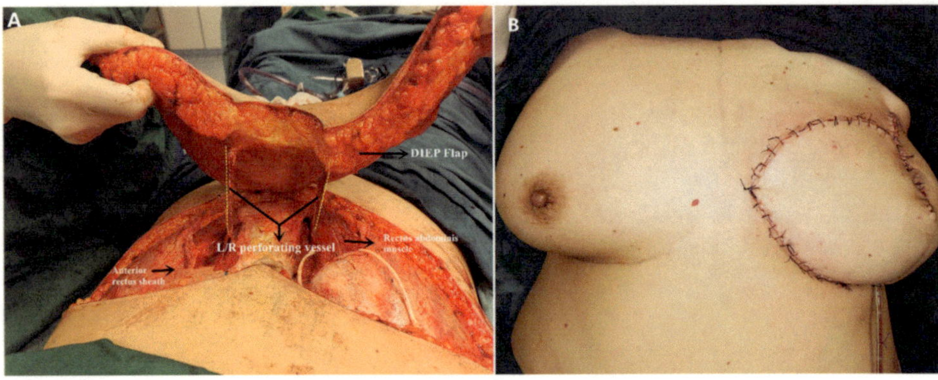

Figure 6.
A panoramic view of DIEP flap and immediate postoperative images.

The choosing of flap perforator vessels and non-invasive anatomy are critical in DIEP surgery. There were, however, substantial variations in the starting position, diameter, and intramuscular course of flap perforator vessels between people or between lateral perforator vessels of the same individual. In traditional surgery, the main perforator is determined by a thorough assessment of each perforator during intraoperative anatomical investigation. The procedure is time-consuming, inefficient, and needs the physician to have extensive personal experience. Furthermore, perforator vessels have a smaller diameter, a wide range of form and location variability, which adds to the complexity and danger of operation [9].

During the development of DIEP flap for more than 30 years, a variety of methods and means for detecting and locating perforator vessels of flap have appeared in clinic. The commonly used methods include: portable ultrasonic Doppler examination: it was first used in 1975 to locate vascular perforator in flap surgery. Its advantages of simple operation, convenient portability and low cost can be used for preliminary vascular evaluation before surgery. However, studies have shown that its high false positive rate reduces the actual clinical guidance value [10]. Color Doppler examination: compared with portable ultrasonic Doppler, color Doppler can provide more detailed hemodynamic information, such as the origin, caliber, intramuscular shape, peak flow rate, resistance index, etc., so as to judge the vascular quality [11]. At present, it has been reported in the literature that color Doppler can detect perforator vessels with a diameter of about 0.7 mm, with an accuracy comparable to that of CTA. If combined with contrast-enhanced ultrasound examination, the effect of vascular development can be further improved [12]. High-resolution magnetic resonance angiography (MRA) examination, conventional MRA resolution is low, although with the emergence of high-resolution MRI and corresponding sequences, MRA can display perforator vessels with a diameter of 1 mm, and can even partially replace CTA examination, but its economy, practicability and scanning time are worth considering [13]. CTA examination: In 2006, Masia et al. [14] first used CTA to locate the inferior abdominal perforator vessel before surgery and selected the dominant perforator for breast reconstruction, and the imaging consistency rate of CTA reached 100%. CTA can provide accurate anatomical information on the perforating point, number, caliber and course of the perforating vessel of DIEP flap. Compared with other examinations, CTA is not susceptible to the influence of the patient's body type, vascular variation and deformity.

At present, CTA imaging technology is more and more widely used in the field of flap repair abroad, especially in the application of abdominal DIEP flap for breast reconstruction after breast cancer surgery [15–17]. However, there are few domestic reports on the clinical application of CTA in delayed breast reconstruction after breast cancer surgery. In traditional DIEP breast reconstruction surgery, the perforator is usually evaluated by color Doppler. However, the accuracy of perforator localization is affected by false positive ultrasonography and operator's subjectivity to some extent. With the wide application of imaging technology, CTA can clearly display the anatomical information of perforator vessels with a diameter > 0.3 mm before surgery. As a "rehearsal" before surgery, surgeons can accurately conduct preoperative clinical operation simulation according to the picture [7]. In recent years, our center has conducted preoperative imaging evaluation for patients who plan to undergo delayed DIEP breast reconstruction. Combined with the different imaging evaluation methods in our hospital before and after 2018, this paper attempts to analyze the application value of CTA in delayed DIEP breast reconstruction surgery.

As a non-invasive, rapid, high image resolution, high accuracy and high specificity preoperative perforator vessel imaging method, CTA examination has been widely used in preoperative localization of perforator vessels of DIEP flap [15, 18]. In this study, we compared baseline data, intraoperative observed indicators, and incidence of postoperative complications between the CTA group and the US group. Among them, the CTA group was significantly better than the preoperative ultrasound localization group in choosing the time of perforator and the anatomic time of perforator. The time required to obtain the same mass flap was significantly shorter in CTA group than in ultrasound group ($p < 0.001$). This conclusion is consistent with most foreign studies [5, 6, 15]. All CTA data in this experiment were identified and read DICOM files by the surgeon himself through HOROS software in the mobile phone or computer. It can objectively evaluate and locate the number of perforator vessels before surgery, and perform a good preoperative operation simulation. At the same time, it is convenient for preoperative communication between doctors and patients, and can also play a positive role in promoting scientific research and teaching. On the other hand, CTA examination can get rid of the dependence of clinical surgeons on radiologists to a certain extent. Previous studies have shown that the agreement between surgeons and radiologists is 67.3%, and surgeons have higher accuracy of preoperative perforator localization [3, 17, 19].

In all cases of CTA, the surgeon can read, measure, draw and mark the intended surgical treatment cases anytime and anywhere in advance, regardless of the limitation of time and space, which is especially convenient for the formulation of remote consultation surgery plans for clinicians. In the CTA group, the operation time and cost can be saved when the skin flap is obtained. According to the study of Haddock et al. [3], compared with the group without preoperative CTA, the time to obtain the flap and the total operation time were longer. However, in the comparison of total operation time in this study, there was no significant statistical difference between the CTA group and the US group. Analysis of this reason may be due to: First, this study was bounded by time nodes. From January 2016 to January 2018, the perforator vessel was evaluated by ultrasonic localization, and from January 2018 to January 2021, the perforator vessel was evaluated by CTA. In the early stage (US group), the operator team paid more attention to the flap resection process. With the further improvement of surgical skills and surgical instruments, surgeons spent more energy on the flap shaping process in the later period (CTA group), which reduced the difference of total operation time between the two groups to a certain extent. Second, 92 cases were included in the US group and 206 in the CTA group in this study. The mismatch in the number of cases may bias the experimental results to a certain extent. In addition, the results of this study indicated that, in the comparison of total operating time between the CTA group and the US group, the mean net operating time of the CTA group was shortened by 34 min. Although it did not translate into statistical *P* value difference, different results may occur with the matching or increasing of the number of cases. Third, in this study, the CTA group contained more patients with double pedicle reconstruction than the US group (58.7 vs. 56.5%), which increased the operation time to a certain extent. In addition, the preoperative evaluation of color Doppler ultrasound in the control group has a certain guiding value for the localization of perforator branches.

The presence of scar in previous abdominal surgery may affect the effect of DIEP flap reconstruction, because scar tissue may affect the normal distribution of blood supply in the abdominal flap, and in severe cases affect the normal shape of perforator vessels, thus increasing the difficulty of surgical anatomy [20, 21]. However, preoperative CTA examination can clearly show the integrity and shape of the deep vessels and perforator vessels under the abdominal wall, which is of greater reference value for patients with surgical history. The present study was stratified according to whether there was a history of accompanying abdominal surgery. The results showed that: for patients with a history of abdominal surgery, the time of flap resection and total operation time in CTA group were lower than those in US group ($P < 0.05$). For patients with no history of abdominal surgery, the time of flap resection in CTA group was lower than that in US group ($P < 0.05$), and there was no significant difference in total operation time ($P > 0.05$). Therefore, it is of great significance to strengthen preoperative CTA examination for patients with a history of abdominal surgery.

In the comparison of postoperative complications between the two groups, 92 patients in the US group had complete necrosis of the skin flap, and 206 patients in the CTA group had all survived. Although the difference between the two groups was not statistically significant, the CTA group may have a higher flap survival rate. To this end, we again compared the rate of secondary surgical exploration between the two groups, the US group was 13.04% (12/92) and the CTA group was 2.91% (6/206), the difference was statistically significant ($P < 0.001$), and CTA could reduce the risk of secondary surgical exploration to a certain extent. As for the consistency comparison between the intraoperative perforator and the dominant perforator evaluated based on imaging data, the consistency rate of imaging surgery was 97.09% (200/206) in the CTA group and 43.48% (40/92) in the US group, the difference was statistically significant ($P < 0.001$). Therefore, CTA examination can more accurately select, measure and locate the dominant perforator before surgery.

CTA examination is not only limited to the application of perforating branches of abdominal flaps, but also can further evaluate the conditions of blood vessels in the chest receiving area (internal arteriovenous) during the preoperative thoracoabdominal joint examination. Especially for some patients with radiation ulcers, reasonable selection of blood vessels in the receiving area can further increase the probability of successful surgery [22]. In addition, in some patients with a history of abdominal surgery, CTA can be better used to evaluate the conditions of abdominal perforator vessels, so as to guide the selection of surgical methods. However, as with any form of imaging, preoperative CTAs are inevitably subject to unexpected findings. Literature reported that the incidence of accidental discovery was 13–75% in CTA studies on DIEP flap program [16]. Wagner et al. suggested that among the 350 patients who met the criteria, 56.9% of the patients found lung nodules and abdominal diseases without special intervention in preoperative imaging examination, 12.9% of the patients received additional imaging examination, and 4.0% of the patients received additional intervention, such as puncture biopsy of lung tumors. In addition, abdominal CTA examination is conducive to the selection of donor skin flap during breast reconstruction surgery, and preoperative CTA evaluation is especially important for patients who plan to undergo SIEA skin flap operation [23, 24]. However, CTAs also have some disadvantages: patients need to be exposed to radiation, which may trigger a certain risk of cancer; In addition, the use of iodine contrast media may cause a small number of people allergic reactions, kidney damage and other unpredictable unexpected conditions.

In summary, CTA technology can accurately provide detailed anatomical information of perforator vessels, facilitate surgical design, reduce intraoperative perforator selection and dissection time, reduce the risk of secondary surgical exploration, and have a high imaging and surgical consistency rate, especially for patients with a history of abdominal surgery, CTA is of higher value. Therefore, CTA examination is worthy of clinical application in delayed DIEP breast flap reconstruction.

6. Conclusions

In delayed DIEP flap breast reconstruction, CTA can significantly shorten the choice time of flap perforation and anatomy time, reduce the risk of secondary surgical exploration and has a high rate of image surgery consistency, which can effectively guide the operation.

Acknowledgements

Xu yuanbing: thesis design, writing, modification, and data proofreading, Pan dai: imagine data measurement and statistics, paper revision, Xu hua: thesis design and revision. The author(s) read and approved the final manuscript. This work was supported by funding from a special fund in the field of major health of the Science and Technology Department of Hubei Province (2022BCE041) and the Natural Science Foundation of Xiaogan City (XGKJ2022010006).

Conflict of interest

The copyright of this academic study belongs to the "Chinese Journal of Cancer." We thank the editor and reviewers of the Journal for their guidance and assistance in the Chinese submission. The English version is the translation of the Chinese version. Please point out if there are any improper points.

Acronyms and abbreviations

DIEP	deep inferior epigastric perforator
CTA	computed tomography angiography
BMI	body mass index
NAS	non-abdominal surgery
MRA	magnetic resonance angiography

Author details

Xu Yuanbing[1*], Pan Dai[2] and Xu Hua[3]

1 Department of Thyroid and Breast Surgery, Xiaogan Hospital Affiliated to Wuhan University of Science and Technology, Xiaogan, Hubei, China

2 Department of Ultrasound, Xiaogan Hospital Affiliated to Wuhan University of Science and Technology, Xiaogan, Hubei, China

3 Department of Plastic Surgery, Shanghai Ninth People's Hospital, Shanghai Jiao Tong University School of Medicine, Shanghai, China

*Address all correspondence to: 443430731@qq.com

IntechOpen

© 2023 The Author(s). Licensee IntechOpen. This chapter is distributed under the terms of the Creative Commons Attribution License (http://creativecommons.org/licenses/by/3.0), which permits unrestricted use, distribution, and reproduction in any medium, provided the original work is properly cited.

References

[1] Liu C, Zhao Z, Gu X, et al. Establishment and verification of a bagged-trees-based model for prediction of sentinel lymph node metastasis for early breast cancer patients. Frontiers in Oncology. 2019;**16**(9):282. DOI: 10.3389/fonc.2019.00282

[2] Yang BL, Ren GS, Song EW, et al. Current status and factors influencing surgical options for breast cancer in China: A nationwide cross-sectional survey of 110 hospitals. The Oncologist. 2020;**25**(10):e1473-e1480. DOI: 10.1634/theoncologist.2020-0001

[3] Haddock NT, Dumestre DO, Teotia SS. Efficiency in DIEP flap breast reconstruction: The real benefit of computed tomographic angiography imaging. Plastic and Reconstructive Surgery. 2020;**146**(4):719-723. DOI: 10.1097/PRS.0000000000007148

[4] Smit JM, Dimopoulou A, Liss AG, et al. Preoperative CT angiography reduces surgery time in perforator flap reconstruction. Journal of Plastic, Reconstructive & Aesthetic Surgery. 2009;**62**(9):1112-1117. DOI: 10.1016/j.bjps.2007.12.090

[5] Tong WM, Dixon R, Ekis H, et al. The impact of preoperative CT angiography on breast reconstruction with abdominal perforator flaps. Annals of Plastic Surgery. 2012;**68**(5):525-530. DOI: 10.1097/SAP.0b013e31823b69a4

[6] Sandberg LJ. Tracing: A simple interpretation method for the DIEP flap CT angiography to help operative decision-making. Plastic and Reconstructive Surgery—Global Open. 2020;**8**(11):e3218. DOI: 10.1097/GOX.0000000000003218

[7] Rozen WM, Bhullar HK, Hunter-Smith D. How to assess a CTA of the abdomen to plan an autologous breast reconstruction. Gland Surgery. 2019;**8**(Suppl 4):S291-S296. DOI: 10.21037/gs.2019.04.10

[8] Wilkins EG, Hamill JB, Kim HM, et al. Complications in postmastectomy breast reconstruction: One-year outcomes of the mastectomy reconstruction outcomes consortium (MROC) study. Annals of Surgery. 2018;**267**(1):164-170. DOI: 10.1097/SLA.0000000000002033

[9] DellaCroce FJ, DellaCroce HC, Blum CA, et al. Myth-busting the DIEP flap and an introduction to the abdominal perforator exchange (APEX) breast reconstruction technique: A single-surgeon retrospective review. Plastic and Reconstructive Surgery. 2019;**143**(4):992-1008. DOI: 10.1097/PRS.0000000000005484

[10] Khan UD, Miller JG. Reliability of handheld Doppler in planning local perforator-based flaps for extremities. Aesthetic Plastic Surgery. 2007;**31**(5):521-525. DOI: 10.1007/s00266-007-0072-9

[11] Kehrer A, Heidekrueger PI, Lonic D, et al. High-resolution ultrasound-guided perforator mapping and characterization by the microsurgeon in lower limb reconstruction. Journal of Reconstructive Microsurgery. 2021;**37**(1):75-82. DOI: 10.1055/s-0040-1702162

[12] Su W, Lu L, Lazzeri D, et al. Contrast-enhanced ultrasound combined with three-dimensional reconstruction in preoperative perforator flap planning. Plastic and Reconstructive Surgery. 2013;**131**(1):80-93. DOI: 10.1097/PRS.0b013e3182729e9e

[13] Rozen WM, Garcia-Tutor E, Alonso-Burgos A, et al. Planning and optimising DIEP flaps with virtual surgery: The Navarra experience. Journal of Plastic, Reconstructive & Aesthetic Surgery. 2010;**63**(2):289-297. DOI: 10.1016/j.bjps.2008.10.007

[14] Masia J, Clavero JA, Larrañaga JR, et al. Multidetector-row computed tomography in the planning of abdominal perforator flaps. Journal of Plastic, Reconstructive & Aesthetic Surgery. 2006;**59**(6):594-599. DOI: 10.1016/j.bjps.2005.10.024

[15] Teunis T, Heerma van Voss MR, Kon M, et al. CT-angiography prior to DIEP flap breast reconstruction: A systematic review and meta-analysis. Microsurgery. 2013;**33**(6):496-502. DOI: 10.1002/micr.22119

[16] Wagner RD, Doval AF, Mehra NV, et al. Incidental findings in CT and MR angiography for preoperative planning in DIEP flap breast reconstruction. Plastic and Reconstructive Surgery—Global Open. 2020;**8**(10):e3159. DOI: 10.1097/GOX.0000000000003159

[17] Weum S, Mercer JB, de Weerd L. Evaluation of dynamic infrared thermography as an alternative to CT angiography for perforator mapping in breast reconstruction: A clinical study. BMC Medical Imaging. 2016;**16**(1):43. DOI: 10.1186/s12880-016-0144-x

[18] Thimmappa N, Bhat AP, Bishop K, et al. Preoperative cross-sectional mapping for deep inferior epigastric and profunda artery perforator flaps. Cardiovascular Diagnosis and Therapy. 2019;**9** (Suppl. 1):S131-S142. DOI: 10.21037/cdt.2018.10.03

[19] Suffee T, Pigneur F, Rahmouni A, et al. Best choice of perforator vessel in autologous breast reconstruction: Virtual reality navigation vs radiologist analysis. A prospective study. Journal of Plastic Surgery and Hand Surgery. 2015;**49**(6):333-338. DOI: 10.3109/2000656X.2015.1053395

[20] Parrett BM, Caterson SA, Tobias AM, et al. DIEP flaps in women with abdominal scars: Are complication rates affected? Plastic and Reconstructive Surgery. 2008;**121**(5):1527-1531. DOI: 10.1097/PRS.0b013e31816b14a5

[21] Roostaeian J, Yoon AP, Sanchez IS, et al. The effect of prior abdominal surgery on abdominally based free flaps in breast reconstruction. Plastic and Reconstructive Surgery. 2014;**133**(3):247e-255e. DOI: 10.1097/01.prs.0000438059.52128.8c

[22] Malhotra A, Chhaya N, Nsiah-Sarbeng P, et al. CT-guided deep inferior epigastric perforator (DIEP) flap localization—better for the patient, the surgeon, and the hospital. Clinical Radiology. 2013;**68**(2):131-138. DOI: 10.1016/j.crad.2012.06.105

[23] Henry FP, Butler DP, Wood SH, et al. Predicting and planning for SIEA flap utilisation in breast reconstruction: An algorithm combining pre-operative computed tomography analysis and intra-operative angiosome assessment. Journal of Plastic, Reconstructive & Aesthetic Surgery. 2017;**70**(6):795-800. DOI: 10.1016/j.bjps.2017.03.011

[24] Cho MJ, Haddock NT, Teotia SS. Clinical decision making using CTA in conjoined, bipedicled DIEP and SIEA for unilateral breast reconstruction. Journal of Reconstructive Microsurgery. 2020;**36**(4):241-246. DOI: 10.1055/s-0039-3400542

Chapter 10

Robotic Technologies in the Treatment of Breast Cancer

Gurami Elgudzhaevich Kvetenadze, E.V. Shivilov, K.S. Arslanov, K.A. Anichkina, L.G. Zhukova and I.E. Khatkov

Abstract

In recent years, there has been a tendency to reduce the volume of surgical intervention in breast cancer in full compliance with the requirements of oncologic radicalism. The abandonment of aggressive surgical treatment, used for many years, is explained, first of all, by the significant success of early diagnosis of breast cancer and the natural increase in the number of patients with early stages of the disease. Robot-assisted radical subcutaneous mastectomy with single-stage endoprosthesis proved to be a feasible and safe method. In all known studies, the surgery has a low conversion rate, a reasonable learning curve and a low complication rate. This technique allows to obtain excellent esthetic results.

Keywords: breast cancer, reconstruction, robotic technology, plastic surgery, breast reconstruction

1. Introduction

Over recent years, there has been a tendency to reduce the volume of surgical intervention in breast cancer in full compliance with the requirements of oncological radicalism. The rejection of aggressive surgical treatment, which has been used for many years, is primarily due to the significant success of early diagnosis of breast cancer and a natural increase in the number of patients with early stages of the disease [1, 2]. At the same time, breast-conserving surgery (BCS) at the initial stages of the disease is recognized as the preferred type of surgical treatment in the vast majority of cases [3, 4]. An important stage in the treatment of early stages of breast cancer should be the unification of the principles of BCS with elements of plastic surgery and precision endovideosurgical techniques. By virtue of the use of modern technologies and improved visualization of the surgical area, the accuracy of surgical manipulations increases and the volume of damaged tissues decreases, thereby minimizing the risk of hematogenic and lymphogenic dissemination [1–4]. In recent decades, the use of robotic technologies in various fields of modern surgery has had a significant impact on surgical technique and patient treatment outcomes. Presently robot-assisted surgery is considered one of the most relevant options for performing prostatectomy, cystectomy, hysterectomy, and is also successfully used in colorectal surgery [5, 6]. Despite the absence of a natural cavity necessary for endoscopic control, robotic interventions have also been used in the surgical treatment of diseases of superficially located organs (thyroid gland), as well as in plastic and reconstructive surgical interventions (oropharyngeal zone and breast) [7].

A patient with histologically verified stages I-IIa breast cancer, who was being treated in the oncosurgical department of the breast of the Loginov Moscow Clinical Scientific Center MHD, underwent a robot-assisted radical subcutaneous mastectomy with single-step endoprosthesis (**Table 1**).

On the eve of the operation, a preoperative cutaneous marking of the area of the alleged tissue dissection with a skin marker is performed (**Figure 1**).

The basic kit for accomplishment robot-assisted subcutaneous mastectomy includes a monitor, a video camera, a light source and a light guide, a 0-degree 10-mm endoscope, a radiofrequency scalpel, three 12-mm trocars, a monopolar endoscopic clamp, an irrigation-aspiration system, a CO_2 insufflator, a "SI Da Vinci Robotic" platform, a bipolar endoscopic clamp, endoscopic monopolar curved scissors (**Figure 2**).

One of the most important issues of the robot-assisted subcutaneous mastectomy is the optimal positioning of the patient's trunk, upper limb and the robot platform in the operating room. At the same time, it is necessary to achieve the most effective interaction of the operating team and avoid the separation of the operating zone by the sleeves and diaphragm of the robotic complex. To achieve all the above-stated goals, the patient should be under general anesthesia with orotracheal intubation in a supine position, the patient's arm on the side of the operation is bent at the elbow joint and put behind the head—this position is ideal both for avoiding conflicts with the robot diagram and for preventing damage because of distortion the brachial plexus. In addition, the introduction of 3 trocars provides effective triangulation of operational equipment in each area of the operative field, which, in return, allows optimizing the location of the elements of the robotic complex. The surgical table is given a slight tilt towards the affected breast. 3 trocars are inserted along the lateral edge of the breast (along the anterior axillary line) at the level of 3–6 ribs (**Figure 3**).

Therefore, the surgeon is located in front of the main console, controlling the robotic complex and other operating equipment, and the assistant is at the surgical table, controlling the movements of the robotic manipulators. The first port is

Indications for performing RARSM	Contraindications to performing RARSM
Age from 35 to 60 years old	Presence of clinically significant comorbidities
Absence of distant and regional metastases	Body mass index less than 24 kg/m^2
The largest tumor size is less than 3 cm	Data on alcohol, drug, and tobacco abuse
Absence of clinical and morphological data on multicentric growth of breast cancer	Breast ptosis of degree 2 (or more)
Absence of clinical and morphological evidence of widespread intraductal invasion	Breast volume is less than 150 and more than 350 cm^3
No clinical or morphological evidence of tumor or inflammatory infiltration and erosion of the skin or nipple	Radiation therapy on the anterior chest wall area on the surgical side
Location of the tumor at least 1.5 cm from the areola	
Breast volume from 150 to 350 cm^3	

Table 1.
Indications and contraindications for performing RARSM.

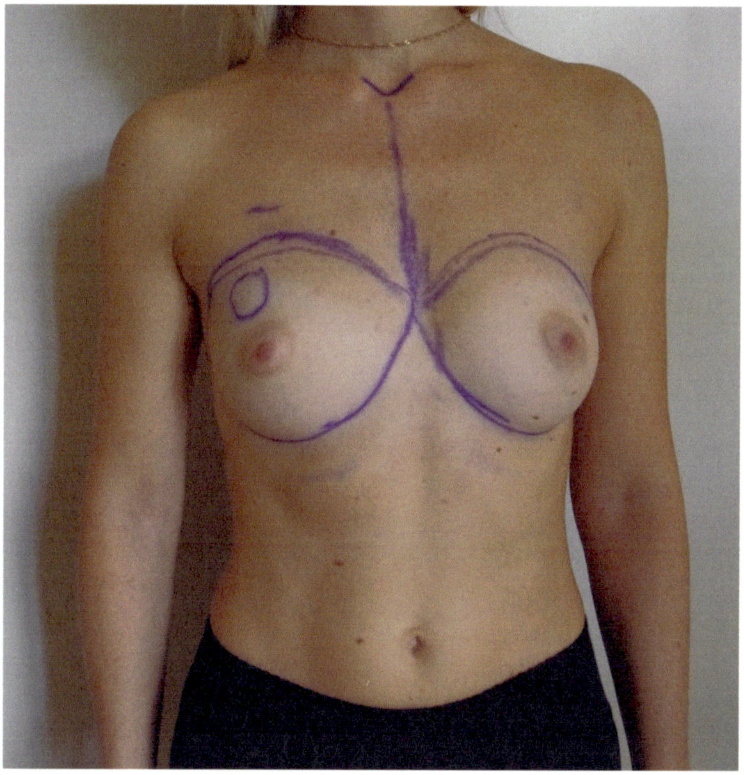

Figure 1.
Preoperative marking (the skin marker indicates the areas of the alleged dissection of the tissues of the right breast, the projection of the tumor on the skin, the median line and the spot of the left breast are indicated).

installed in the axillary region through a two-centimeter discission of the skin at the border of the breast and the axillary region.

A 12-mm trocar is inserted into this port, into which a Meriland clamp is installed. To create a sufficient working space, the required amount of carbon dioxide is dosed through the first port.

Carbon dioxide is insufflated at very low pressure (4–5 mm Hg) to prevent a subcutaneous emphysema. An 8 mm trocar for the endovideosystem is installed in the second port. A 12 mm trocar for Ligasure™ scissors is inserted into the third one (**Figure 4**).

While using ports, there is no need to form a deep and wide subcutaneous nook. In general, it was enough to separate the subcutaneous adipose tissue by no more than 1–2 cm along the entire contour of the skin discission. In addition, constant insufflation of carbon dioxide facilitates surface dissection, promotes stretching of Cooper's ligaments and separation of glandular breast tissue. An additional advantage of this technique is that 3-port access avoids excessive uncontrolled stretching of the edges of the skin, which contributes to better wound healing in the postoperative period and provides an acceptable esthetic result. After insertion of monopolar curved scissors and bipolar clamp, the instruments are docked to the robotic complex. Using the "SI Da Vinci Robotic" system allows to arbitrarily change the position and length of the robotic arms, facilitating work in the very small operative field. In addition, during manipulations, the position of the channels can change independently of each other,

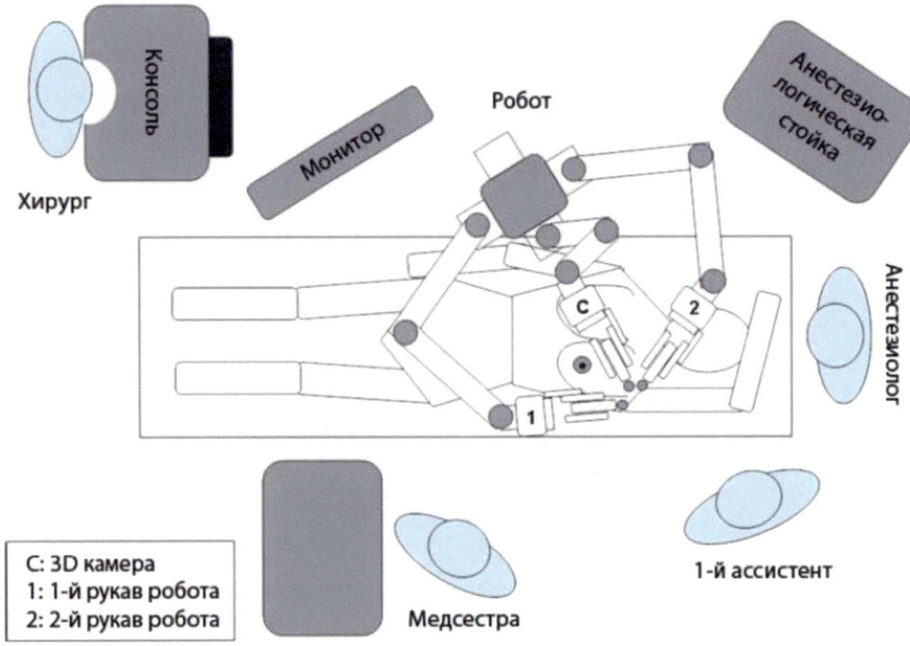

Figure 2.
The layout of the patient on the surgical table, the operating team and the "Da Vinci" complex.

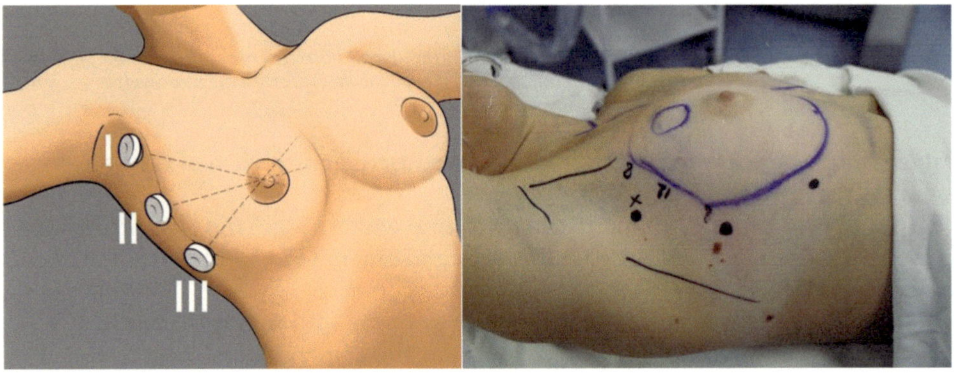

Figure 3.
Location of trocars during left-sided robot–assisted subcutaneous mastectomy: a—schematic representation of trocars; b—marking the location of trocars on the surgical table.

which makes it possible to change the angles of robotic instruments in relation to the operative field. Finally, using such access allows to attach a system for CO_2 insufflation so as to provide the best dissection conditions.

The stages of skin flap formation and dissection of the nipple-areola complex during robot-assisted radical subcutaneous mastectomy basically have the same features as conventional video-assisted mastectomy. Dissection is performed with robotic monopolar scissors and bipolar forceps. During dissection with scissors, the activation time of thermal energy is minimized to prevent thermal damage of the skin flap.

DOI: http://dx.doi.org/10.5772/intechopen.112916

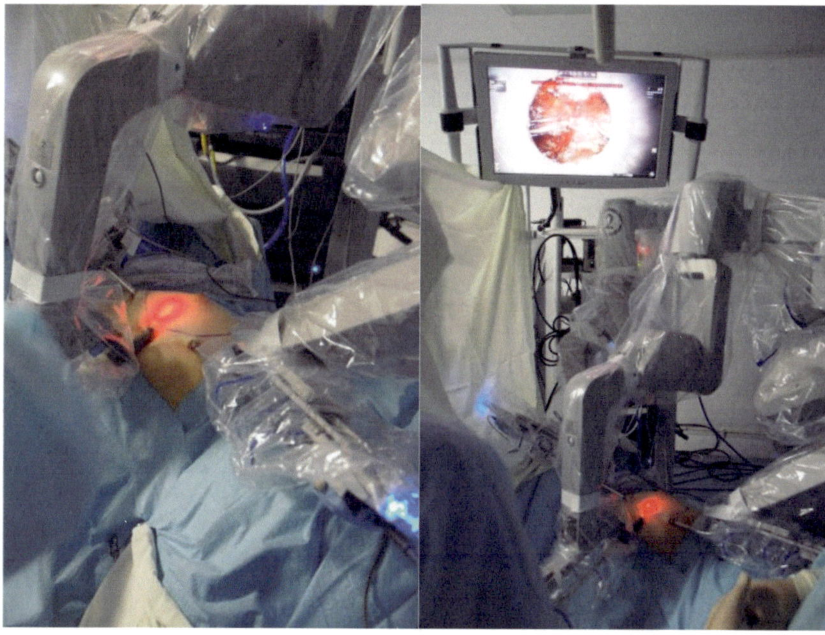

a *b*

Figure 4.
View of the operative field with installed trocars (a) and connected robotic complex (b).

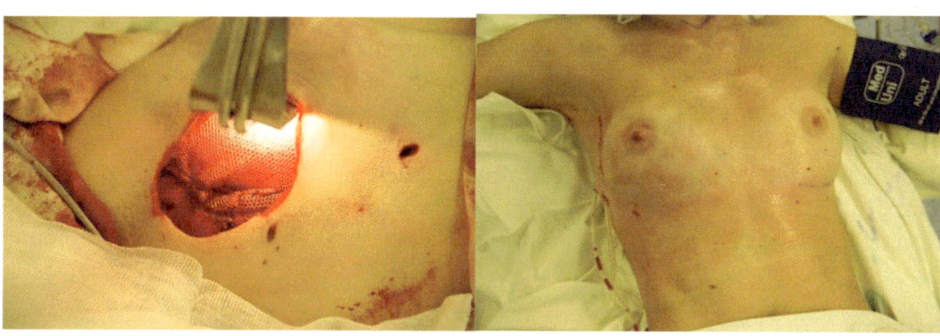

a *b*

Figure 5.
The appearance of the operative field after the installation of the endoprosthesis (a) and the final appearance of the mammary glands after the operation (b).

After the dissection is completed and the glandular breast tissue is completely separated, the robotic complex is disconnected. Then the trocars are removed. A linear discission connects the installation points of I and II trocars and then the breast gross specimen is removed. Lymphodissection of 1–2 levels is performed. Next, to perform the reconstructive stage of the operation, the greater pectoral muscle is separated from the V–VI ribs to the sternum. An anatomical silicone prosthesis is placed under the greater pectoral muscle. A drainage is installed in the muscle nook, which is removed through a skin discission along the inframammary fold, previously used to install the III robotic port. After completion of all manipulations, the surgical wound is sutured with an intradermal suture (**Figure 5**).

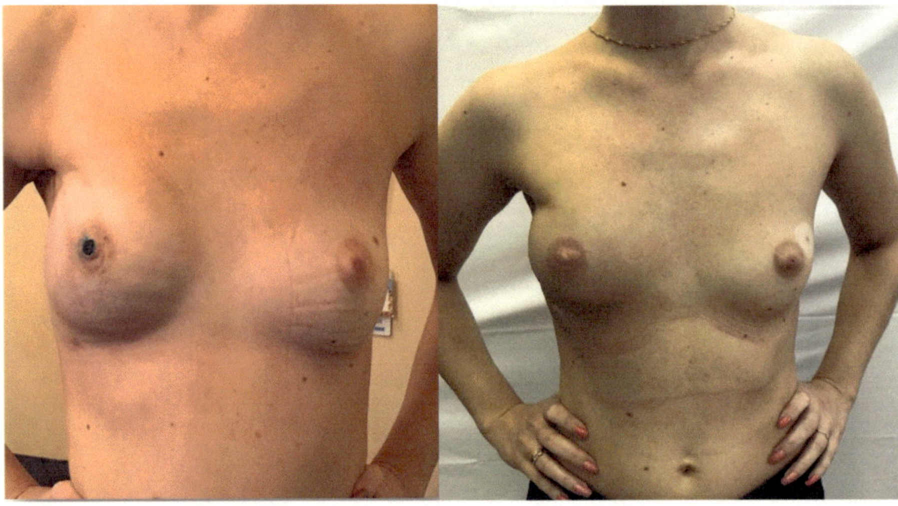

Figure 6.
Appearance of patient a, 35 years old, diagnosed with right breast cancer stage I cT1cN0M0 G2, luminal type a, after performing robot-assisted radical subcutaneous mastectomy with single-step endoprosthesis: a—1 month after surgery; b—1 year after surgery.

2. Results

After performing robot-assisted radical subcutaneous mastectomy with single-step endoprosthesis, the severity of the endoprosthesis folds in the first weeks of the postoperative period is minimal, after 3–4 months, the endoprosthesis folds or pericapsular fluid are not determined by medical ultrasound. Early post-surgery complications did not occur. There was no case of significant pericapsular fibrosis or implant migration after robot-assisted radical subcutaneous mastectomy (**Figure 6**).

3. Discussion

The new Da Vinci SP robotic surgical platform offers many advantages, including better visualization using 3D optics, improved ergonomics of instruments equipped with a high degree of freedom of movement, and a better workspace due to the insufflation used. Discissions for the installation of ports are carried out along the anterior axillary line, which allows to obtain excellent esthetic results. The main disadvantages of this surgical technique include: the duration of the operation, high value, as well as low equipment with robotic installations in medical and preventive treatment centres in the Russian Federation. Robot-assisted radical subcutaneous mastectomy with with single-step endoprosthesis proved to be a feasible and safe method. In all known research studies, the operation has a low conversion rate, a reasonable learning curve and a low level of complications [8, 9]. The authors explain the low frequency of flap necrosis by the location of the discission and better visualization using 3D optics [10]. Oncological results were not reported, since the duration of observation in all research studies was less than 5 years. In all cases, excellent esthetic results were reported, and one study described the degree of patient satisfaction—most were satisfied with the results of the operation, especially in terms of the placement and length of the discission [11].

4. Conclusion

Robot-assisted radical subcutaneous mastectomy is a safe and radical intervention that can be effectively used in the surgical treatment of breast cancer in the early stages of the disease. This technique is associated with a low incidence of early and late complications, and allows to obtain excellent esthetic results.

Author details

Gurami Elgudzhaevich Kvetenadze, E.V. Shivilov*, K.S. Arslanov, K.A. Anichkina, L.G. Zhukova and I.E. Khatkov
SBIH Moscow Clinical Scientific and Practical Center named after A.S. Loginov of DHM, Russia

*Address all correspondence to: ev.shivilov@mknc.ru

IntechOpen

© 2024 The Author(s). Licensee IntechOpen. This chapter is distributed under the terms of the Creative Commons Attribution License (http://creativecommons.org/licenses/by/3.0), which permits unrestricted use, distribution, and reproduction in any medium, provided the original work is properly cited.

References

[1] Volchenko AA, Pak DD. Surgical technologies in the organ-preserving treatment of breast cancer patients. Onkologija. Zhurnal im. P.A. Gercena. 2013;**3**:48-51. (In Russ.)

[2] Kaprin AD, Starinsky VV, Petrova GV, editors. State of oncological care for the Russian population in 2014. M.: P.A. Herzen MNIOI. branch of FGBU "NMIRC" of the Ministry of Health of Russia; 2015. ill. - 236 c. ISBN 978-5-85502-210-0

[3] Zikirjahodzhaev AD, Rasskazova EA. Oncoplastic resections for breast cancer. Onkologija. Zhurnal im. P.A. Gercena. 2015;**4**:80-84. (In Russ.)

[4] Letjagin VP, Grigor'eva TA. Reconstructive plastic surgery in the treatment of breast cancer patients. Opuholi Zhenskoj Reproduktivnoj Sistemy. 2012;**2**:30. (In Russ.)

[5] Kriger AG, Teplov AA, Berelavichus SV, et al. Robot-assisted operations in the pelvic cavity. Hirurgija. Zhurnal im. N.I. Pirogova. 2013;**12**:29-36. (In Russ.)

[6] Fedorov AV, Kriger AG, Berelavichus SV, et al. Robot-assisted operations in abdominal surgery. Hirurgija. Zhurnal im. N.I. Pirogova. 2010;**1**:16-21. (In Russ.)

[7] D'Souza M, Gendreau J, Feng A, et al. Robotic-assisted spine surgery: History, efficacy, cost and future trends. Robotic Surgery. 2019;**6**:9-23. DOI: 10.2147/RSRR.S190720

[8] Lai HW. Robotic nipple-sparing mastectomy and immediate breast reconstruction with gel implant. Annals of Surgical Oncology. 2019;**26**(1):53-54. DOI: 10.1245/s10434-018-6711-3

[9] Houvenaeghel G, Bannier M, Rua S, et al. Breast cancer robotic nipple sparing mastectomy: Evaluation of several surgical procedures and learning curve. World Journal of Surgical Oncology. 2019;**17**(1):27. DOI: 10.1186/s12957-019-1567-y

[10] Sarfati B, Struk S, Leymarie N, et al. Robotic prophylactic nipple-sparing mastectomy with immediate prosthetic breast reconstruction: A prospective study. Annals of Surgical Oncology. 2018;**25**(9):2579-2586. DOI: 10.1245/s10434-018-6555-x

[11] Toesca A, Peradze N, Manconi A, et al. Robotic nipple-sparing mastectomy for the treatment of breast cancer: Feasibility and safety study. Breast. 2017;**31**:51-56. DOI: 10.1016/j.breast.2016.10.009

Chapter 11

Treatment of Symmastia after Breast Reconstruction: Integration of Techniques

Márcia Balbina Lorenzo Hoyos

Abstract

Introduction: Acquired Symmastia (or synmastia) after breast implants is an uncommon complication after breast reconstruction. There are several techniques for correcting this complication, but there is no consensus. Methods: The surgical treatment of three cases of acquired retromuscular symmastia after breast reconstruction are described with the integration of techniques: points of adhesion in the intermammary groove, elevation of the anterior capsule flap with the creation of a neopectoral pocket (precapsular space) and exchange of implants. In two cases, the procedure was associated with fat grafting. Results: The patients evolved well, with correction of the symptoms and were satisfied with the esthetic result. There was no recurrence of the problem, with a follow-up from 9 months to 3 years. Conclusions: It is suggested an integration of techniques for the correction of symmastia (adhesion points and confection of a neopectoral pocket store with anterior capsule flap) after breast reconstruction, which can also be performed in cases of such complication after breast augmentation. This procedure can be associated with fat grafting for esthetic refinement and there may be an improvement in eventual contracture.

Keywords: mastectomy, segmental, surgery, plastic, prostheses and implants, prosthesis implantation, mammaplasty

1. Introduction

Symmastia after breast implants is a rare and highly recurrent complication [1]. The incidence is unknown [2]. In 1983, Symmastia (from Greek syn - together, masto - breast) was defined for the first time as a confluence of the mammary borders through the midline and loss of the intermammary fold [3]. Symmastia can be congenital or acquired, when it is due to the poor positioning of the implants that cross the midline. The first reference for correction of acquired symmastia was in 1988 [4]. The acquired symmastia can be monocapsular (**Figure 1(a)**) (when the implant pocket communicate becoming only one), or bicapsular (**Figure 1(b)**) (when there are two capsules, one or both implants can be medialized and there is a loss of insertion of the midline adhesions) [5]. It is considered severe when both sides of the capsule need to be corrected. When the implants are medialized, but with the medial

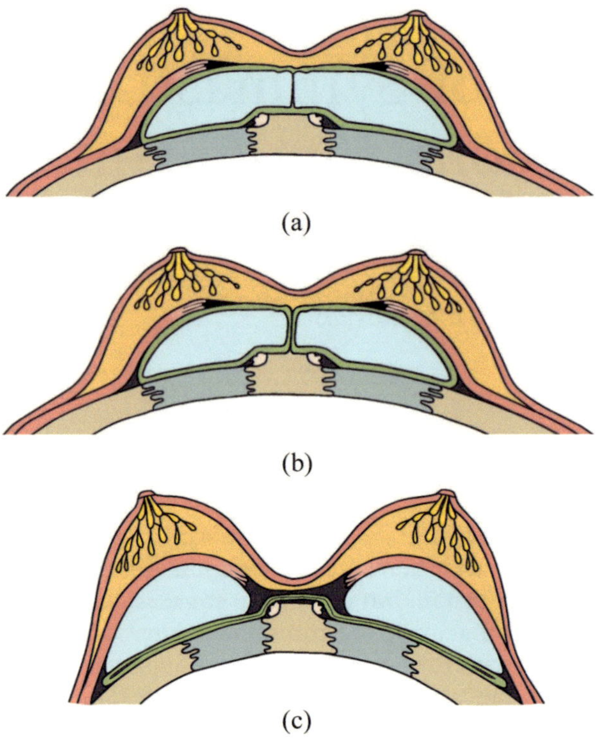

Figure 1.
(a) Representation of retromuscular monocapsular symmastia. (b) Representation of retromuscular bicapsular symmastia. (c) Representation of simasty correction with central membership points and making new retro pectoral pocket.

sternal fascia intact, the term "medial malposition" is preferred [5]. Khan [6] suggests an etiological classification for the types of symmastia (**Table 1**). In this work, we describe three cases of patients with symmastia after breast reconstruction who were treated surgically with an integration of techniques.

Tipo 1	Developmental synmastia. No aberrant communication between the two breasts anterior to the sternum.
Tipo 1a	Idiopathic webbing of cleavage in a small or average-sized breast.
Tipo 1b	Traction synmastia. Webbing seen with mammary hyperplasia.
Tipo 2	Acquired synmastia. Aggressive medial dissection resulting in gradual detachment of presternal skin with underlying communication between the two mammary pockets.
Tipo 2a	Synmastia following subglandular augmentation.
Tipo 2b	Synmastia following submuscular augmentation.
Tipo 3	Synmastia associated with capsular contracture. Medial boundary of the breast is displaced toward the midline without any communication between the two implant pockets.
Tipo 3a	Complete or bilateral, where both medial boundaries are displaced medially and are joined in the middle.
Tipo 3b	Incomplete or unilateral, where medial displacement of the breast has taken place unilaterally.

Table 1.
Khan's etiological classification of symmastia.

2. Objective

To report an integration of techniques for the surgical treatment of symmastia after breast implant reconstruction, also indicated for the treatment of symmastia after breast augmentation.

3. Methods

For the discussion of this report, a bibliographic survey was carried out in the Medline and Cochrane Database, using the descriptors "symmastia", "breast reconstruction" and "surgical treatment". All articles were reviewed, with inclusion only of those that referred to acquired symmastia.

4. Procedure

The patients underwent a surgical procedure under general anesthesia, and all were discharged the next day. Initially, the desired breast furrow was marked with methylene blue, as well as the midline and the inner edge of the breasts to be reconfected.

The prostheses and/or expanders were removed through a scar in the breast crease (previous or not) or by the scar from the mastectomy.

The midline region was scarified with a small curette or electrocautery, followed by adhesion points with non-absorbable threads: at least three points on the midline with 2–0 mononylon, following previous demarcation and a sequence of at least three points for delimitation of the new medial margin of the breasts (on each side of the store).

Then, the anterior capsule flap was made. Decreasing the power of the electrocautery, the anterior capsule of the pectoralis major muscle was detached, which was folded, in order to make a neo pectoral pocket. In two cases, partial capsulectomy was performed and material was sent for anatomopathological examination. The anterior capsule was fixed to the posterior by some points of mononylon 2–0 to close the previous pocket and inferiorly it was fixed with several points on the lower edge of the previous space. This prevented the accumulation of liquids (seroma/hematoma) in the old pocket, as well as sliding movements of the new prosthesis over the previous space. Thus, the previous area was completely closed and the manufactured pocket can be expanded laterally, inferiorly or superiorly, according to the need of each case.

Finally, new breast implants were placed, suction drains were inserted and the usual synthesis of the tissue planes was carried out (**Figure 1(c)**). The drains were removed on an outpatient basis, after 2 to 5 days.

There were no major complications. Patients 1 and 3 required drainage for a longer time due to high blood flow rate, and patient 2 used antibiotics for 2 weeks in the postoperative period, due to a slightly hyperemic irradiated breast.

5. Results

Case 1: Patient operated on 03/15/2017 presenting mono capsular symmastia (previously submitted to bilateral mastectomy in another service, with resection of the areola on the right and resection of inverted T skin on the left; placement of an anatomical expander on the right 450 cc and prosthesis anatomical left of 490 cc textured and evolving at the time with partial necrosis of flaps on the left). Right breast previously irradiated. Symmastia correction was performed (there was complete communication of 6 cm vertically in the pre-sternal region) as described and placement of 455 cc microtextured super high profile prostheses and correction of left breast scars. **Figures 2–5**. There was no recurrence of symmastia, but she evolved with distant and locoregional tumor recurrence on 03/03/2019, and death on 07/2020 **Table 2**.

Case 2: Surgery performed on 23/05/2018. Patient underwent bilateral mastectomy in another service with resection of the nipple areola complex on the right and implant placement - expander prosthesis on the right 460 (Becker 35) and 390 anatomic prosthesis on the left. She presented bicapsular symmastia, separated only by a capsule beam, with complete loss of sternal adhesion. The implants were changed to ultra-high profile round prostheses 590 cc on the right and high profile 450 cc on the left. On that occasion, fat grafting was also performed on the right breast (70 cc). **Figures 6–11**. Subsequently, 120 cc lipografting was performed on the right on 7/7/2019 and the reconstruction of the areomamilar complex (CAM) on 7/2020 was reconstructed. Right breast previously irradiated **Table 2**.

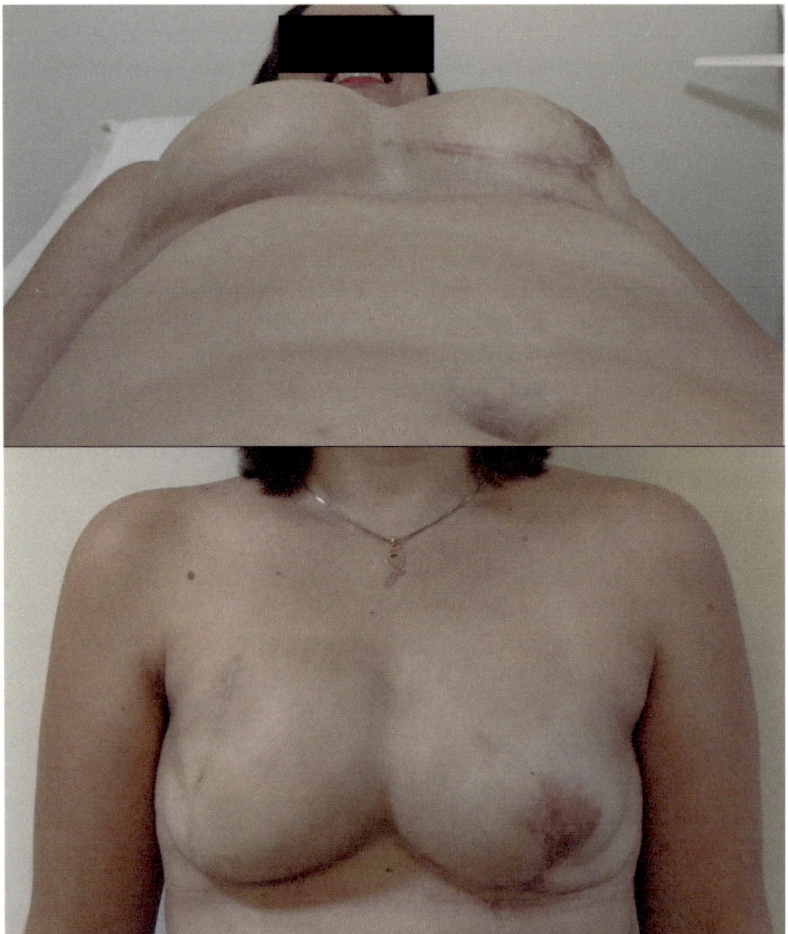

Figure 2.
Case 1: Preoperative.

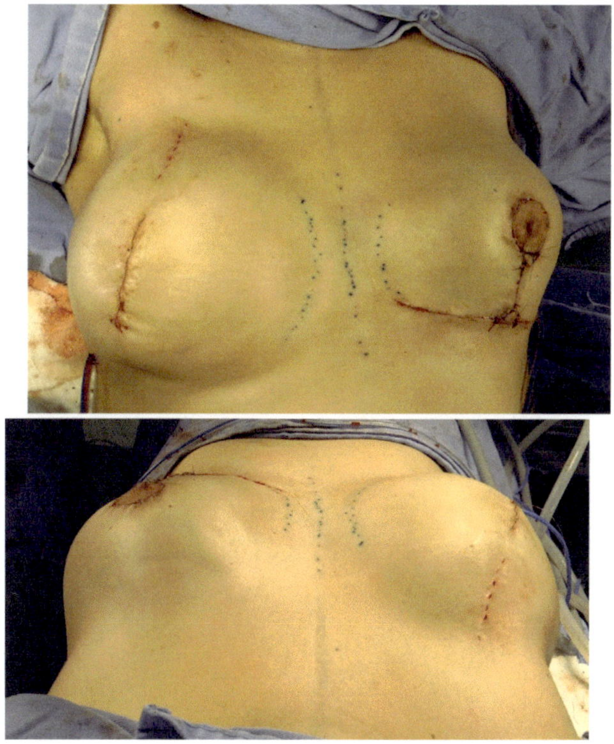

Figure 3.
Case 1: Immediate postoperative period.

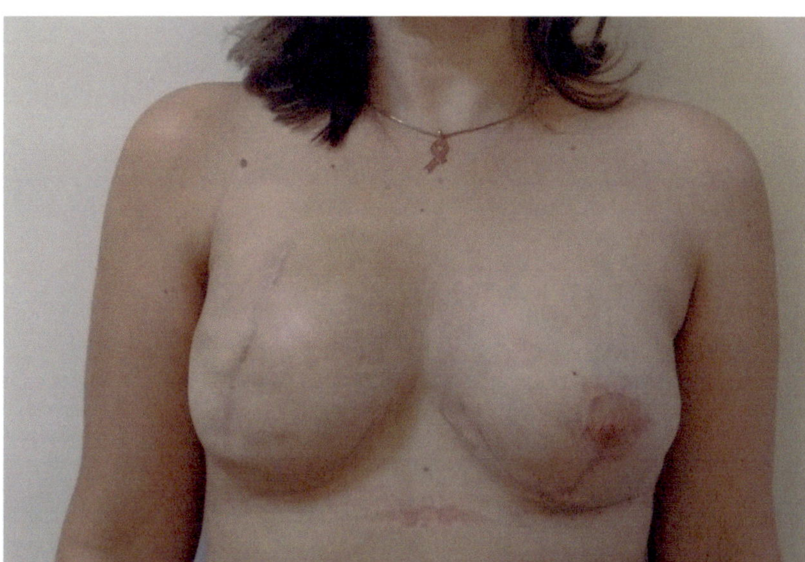

Figure 4.
Case 1: Postoperative 5 months.

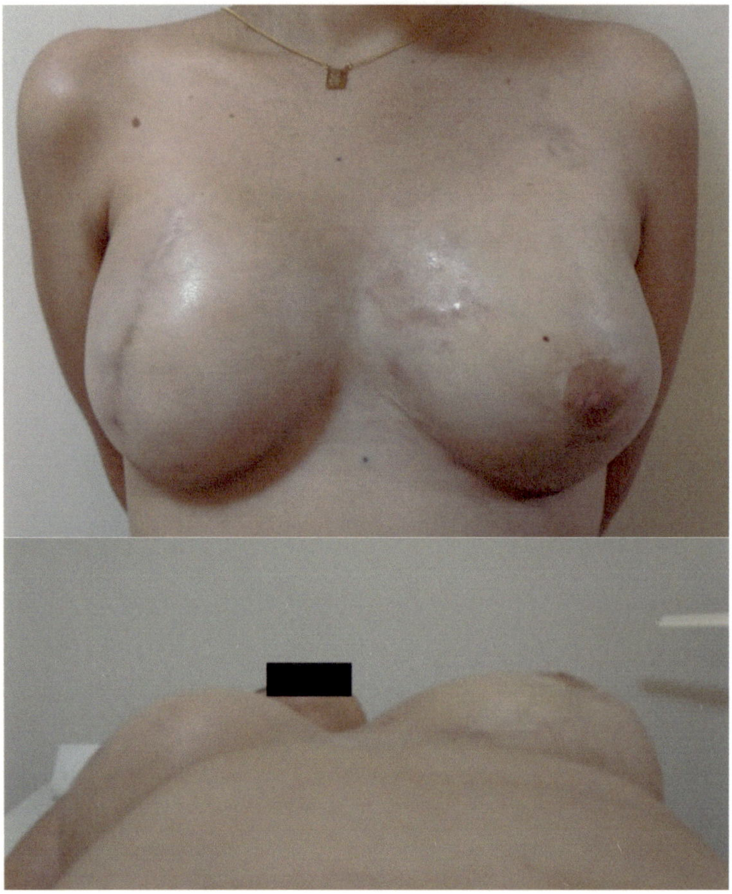

Figure 5.
Case 1: Postoperative 3 years.

Case	Type of retro muscular symmastia	Implants withdrawn from patients with symmastia	Implants placed for the correction of symmastia	Associated fat grafting with the exchange of implants	Anatomopatological capsule
1	Monocapsular	Mentor Texturized anatomic prosthesis 490 cc (left). Mentor texturized anatomic expander 450 cc (right)	Mentor texturized super high profile round prostheses 455 cc	Not done	Right capsule: Fragments exhibiting involvement inflammatory process Focal and discreet fibroplasia. Absence of malignancy

Case	Type of retro muscular symmastia	Implants withdrawn from patients with symmastia	Implants placed for the correction of symmastia	Associated fat grafting with the exchange of implants	Anatomopatological capsule
2	Bicapsular	Mentor Texturized anatomic prothesis 390 cc (left). Mentor texturized anatomic expanding prosthesiis Becker 35,460 cc (right)	Mentor texturized high profile round 450 cc (left) Mentor texturized super high profile round 590 cc (right)	70 cc fat on the right. Not done on the left	Not done
3	Bicapsular	Mentor texturized anatomical prostheses 440 cc	Mentor texturized super high profile round prostheses 450 cc	60 cc fat on the left. 110 cc on the right	Capsules with no lymphocytic proliferation. Absence of malignancy

Table 2.
Summary of cases regarding the type of simastia, implants before and after correction of the problem, association of fat graft during implant replacement and anatomopathological examination of the implant capsule.

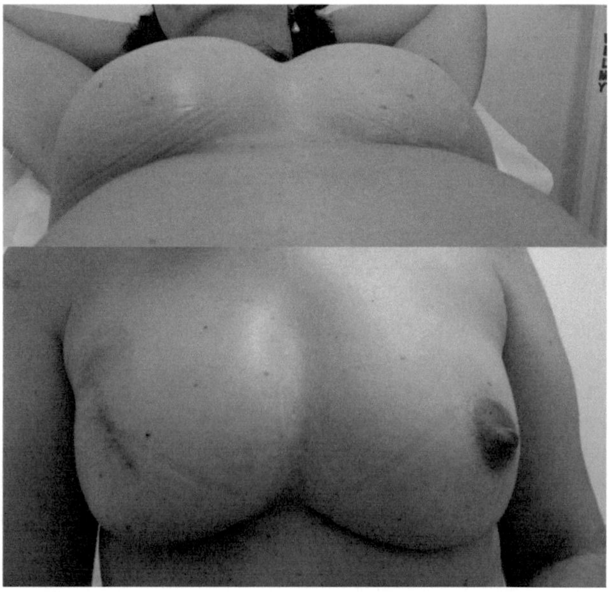

Figure 6.
Case 2: Preoperative.

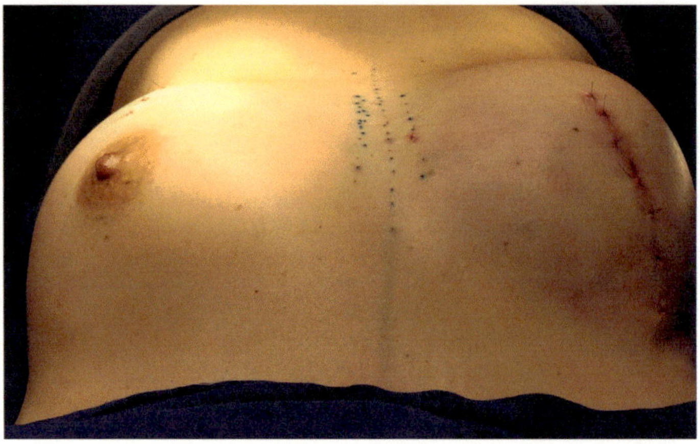

Figure 7.
Case 2: Immediate postoperative period.

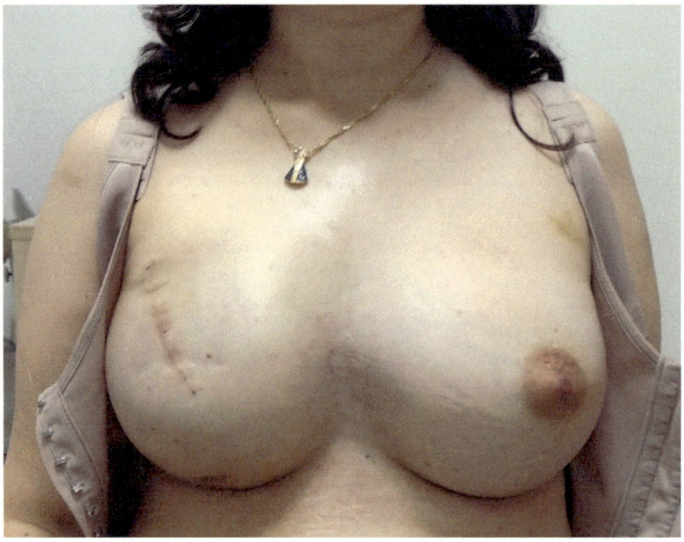

Figure 8.
Case 2: Postoperative 3 weeks.

Case 3: Surgery performed on 06/2020. Patient previously submitted to bilateral mastectomy in another service with resection of the nipple-areola complex on the right and placement of 440 textured anatomical implants. Bicapsular symmastia, separated only by the capsules, and disinsertion of the skin of the pre-sternal region. Correction of symmastia and placement of 455 cc super high profile microtextured round prostheses and fat grafting 110 cc on the right and 60 cc on the left. Subsequently, a new fat graft was performed (40 cc on the right and 30 cc on the left) with reconstruction of the CAM on the right and correction of scars on the left **Figures 12–18** and **Table 2**.

DOI: http://dx.doi.org/10.5772/intechopen.112917

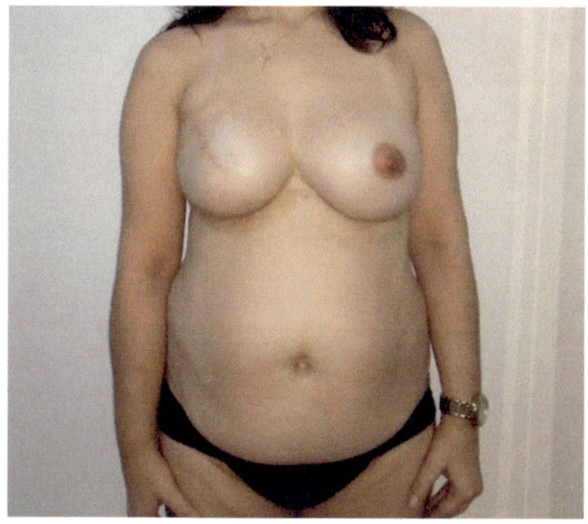

Figure 9.
Case 2: Postoperative 1 year.

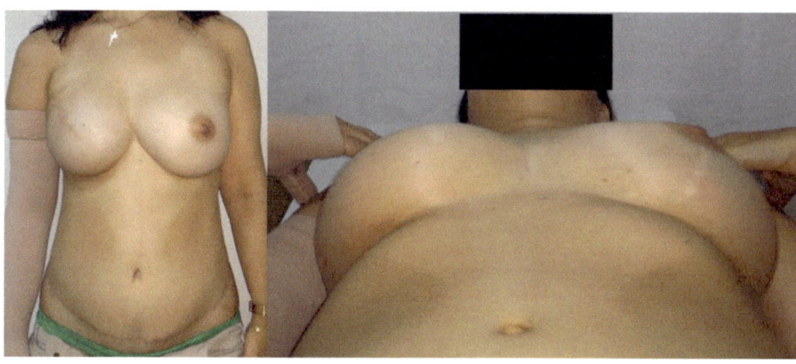

Figure 10.
Case 2: Postoperative period 1 year and 8 months.

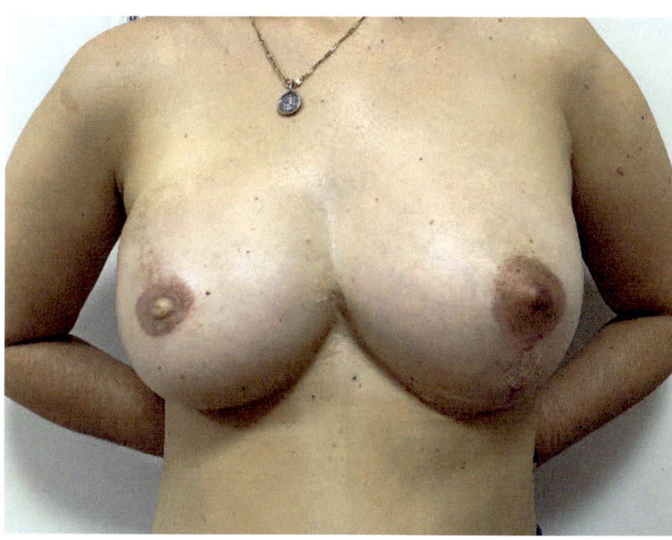

Figure 11.
Case 2: Postoperative 2 years and 6 months.

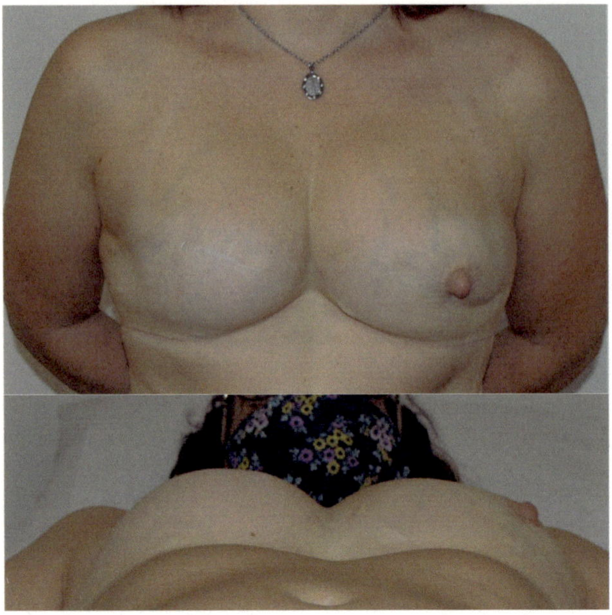

Figure 12.
Case 3: Preoperative.

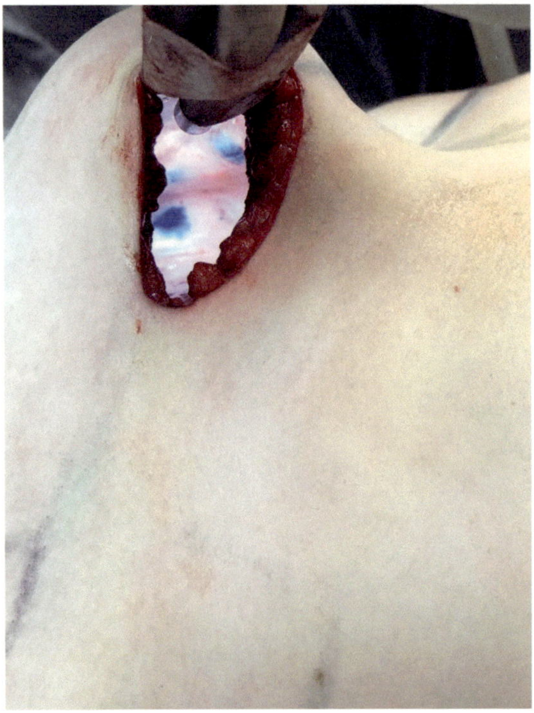

Figure 13.
Case 3: Intraoperative detail: Marking with methylene blue for adhesion points.

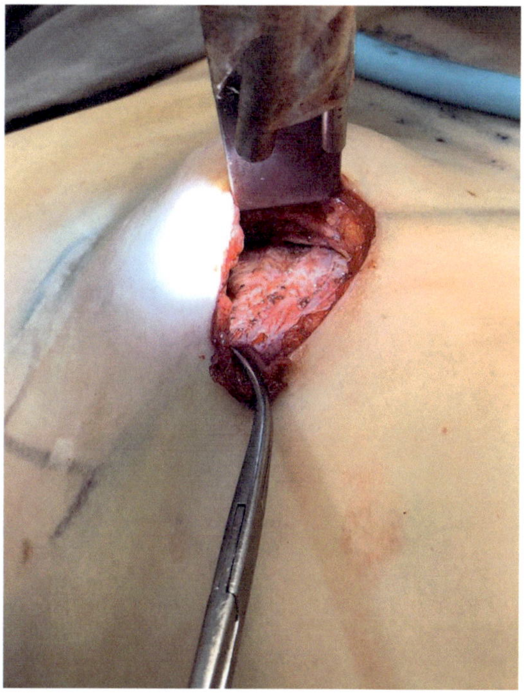

Figure 14.
Case 3: Intraoperative detail: Anterior capsule dissection.

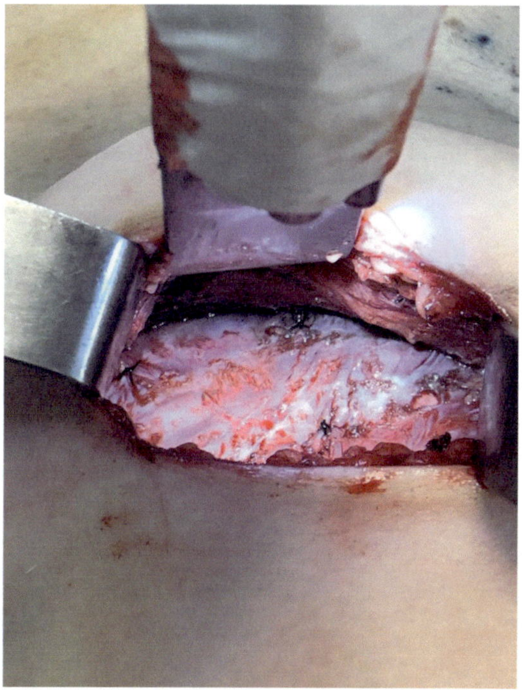

Figure 15.
Case 3: Intraoperative detail of neo retromuscular pocket and anterior capsule attached to the posterior one.

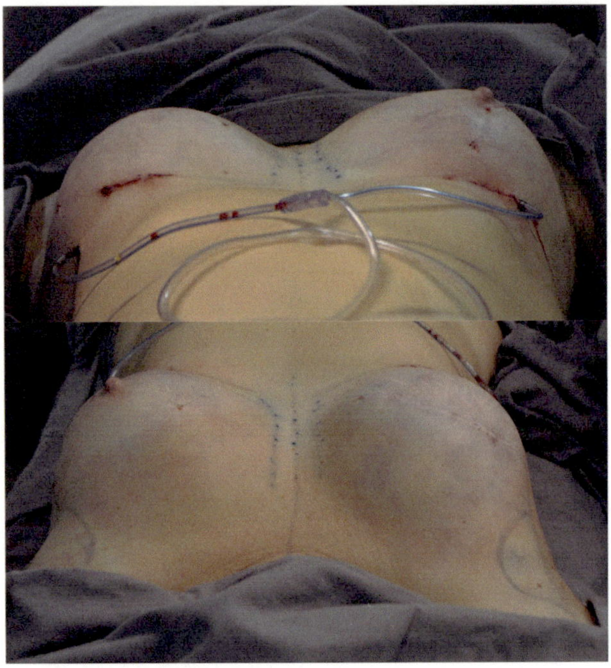

Figure 16.
Case 3: Immediate postoperative period.

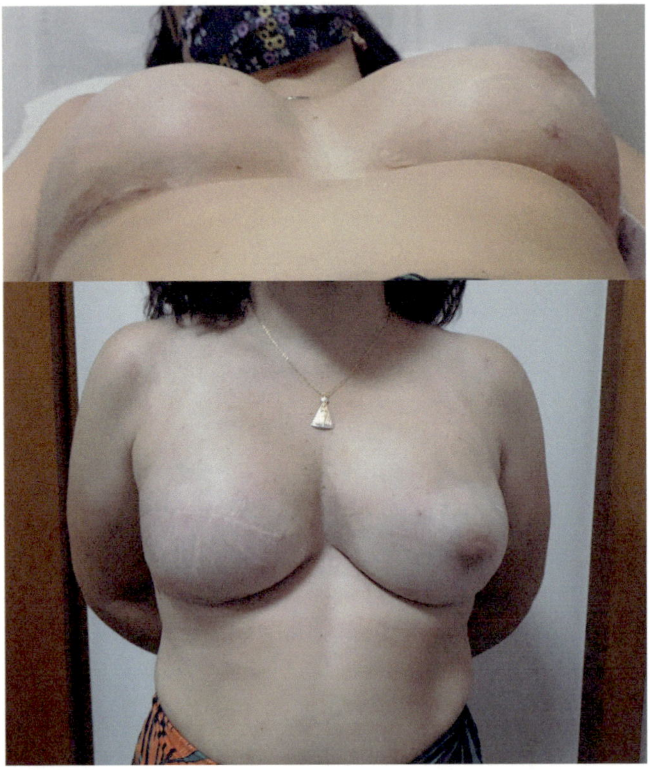

Figure 17.
Case 3: Postoperative 1 month.

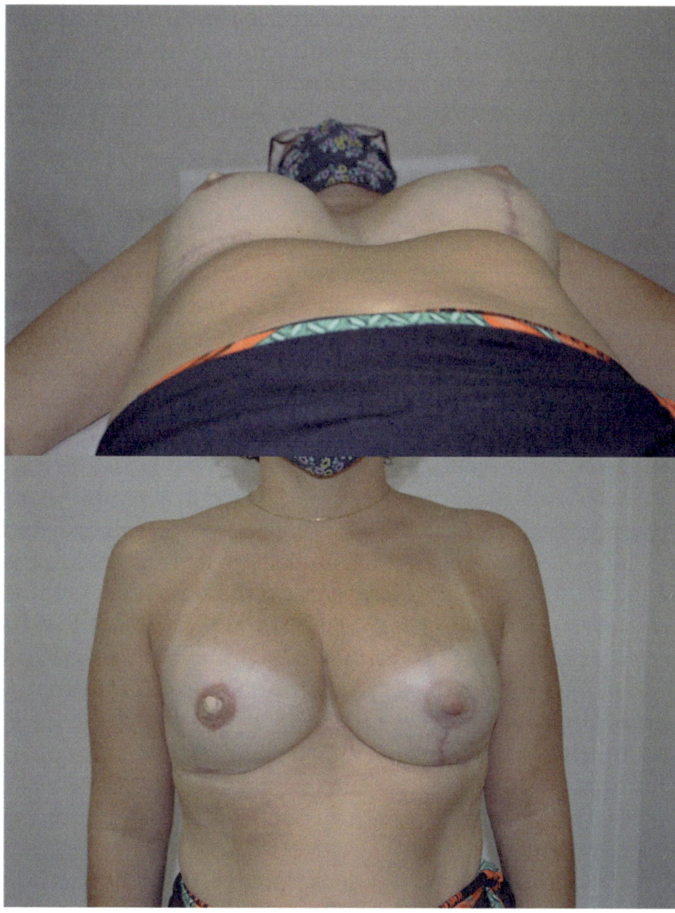

Figure 18.
Case 3: Postoperative 9 months.

6. Discussion

There are not many case series in the literature on correction techniques for symmastia [2] discriminating symmastia after breast reconstruction.

The most likely cause of retropectoral symmastia is exaggerated dissection in the medial region of the breast [2, 7–9]. Other facts can corroborate. Some patients have the insertion of the pectoralis major muscles as thin as 3 to 4 mm at their origin, along the sternum from the 2nd to the 5th ribs, predisposing to this complication after placement of retromuscular implants. A wrong elevation of the pectoralis minor muscle (whose insertion may be less than 1 cm from the insertion of the pectoralis major by 24%, according to anatomical study [10]), with a consequent poor positioning of the implants, would result in a medial force vector for the implant [10, 11]. This fact, added to the excessive medial dissection, with involvement of the internal mammary artery and perivascular fibers, in patients with fine insertion of the pectoralis major muscle would stimulate the sliding of the implants to the midline, with dehiscence of the sternal pectoralis major muscle [11]. However, Hammond [7] disagrees with this because the pectoral muscle would always push the prostheses up and out toward the armpits and basically credits the symmastia to a technical error. In the case of breast reconstruction, the use of expanders could favor the rupture of the medial fibers of the pectoral [12].

Excessive size and/or wide-base implants would also favor symmastia [1, 8, 13].

Recurrence after treatment of symmastia is a common problem [14]. Therefore, the integration of techniques is suggested in this work.

The simple removal of the implants and reconstruction in a second step would be the safest and most simple technique and preferred by some authors [9, 15]. However, this resource is usually left for recurring cases.

Basically, capsulotomy/capsulorrhaphy, sternal dermal adhesions, creation of a new pocket and integration of techniques (including muscle repair and use of dermal matrices) are described for the correction of symmastia [2].

The incision for approaching the implants in this study was the previous mastectomy scar (case 1) or in the breast crease. Scars in the pre-sternal area or intermammary fold must be avoided due to the poor esthetic result and the possibility of keloids [13].

Regarding adhesion techniques, after removing the implants and checking whether the symmastia was mono or bicapsular, the central region (intermammary groove) was scarified, and non-absorbable points were given between the central anterior and posterior capsule and medially to delimit the breasts, similar to Pavelecini et al. [13]. However, differently from these authors, it was decided to create a new pre-capsular space for the implant through the folding of the anterior capsule, maintaining the retropectoral space, to guarantee the correct position of the prostheses. Becker [14], in a series of 5 cases for correction of symmastia, shows only one case after breast reconstruction. It suggests central adhesion in the sternum with non-absorbable threads after anterior and posterior capsulectomy, and use of the same implant store, but with replacement for adjustable implants which were gradually filled in 1 week after surgery. It presents good results, but it is a more expensive technique (due to the use of expanding prostheses).

For the construction of a neopectoral pocket, in the reported cases, the periprosthetic capsules were "mature". Very thin capsules would make it difficult or technically make the procedure impossible, but this is rare [9]. In cases of breast reconstruction, the most usual is a relatively thick capsule, especially in irradiated cases, and this fact allowed the creation of this new retromuscular space, in the described cases, without difficulty. The new implant was repositioned, but there would also have been a contracture correction, as suggested by some authors, if it had previously been so. Furthermore, it also allows the capsules to be studied, as in cases 1 and 3. Creating a new space is technically less difficult and more accurate than trying to reduce the old space with sutures only [9, 16]. It also minimizes trauma and optimizes the size and position of the new space [17]. Changing implants while maintaining the same previous space as symmastia is probably a mistake because it would put greater pressure on the lines of correction sutures [16, 18]. This allowed that, in the reported cases, the implants were increased in size, as the patients requested it. Care was taken to use prostheses with greater projection and smaller diameter. So there was no problem in creating a larger pocket.

Regarding the technique of the neopectoral pocket, the fact that the lateralized muscle is not repaired, which could favor the force vector to push the implant medially [11], has been questioned. However, with the integration of techniques, medial capsulorrhaphy would totally or partially solve this problem.

The inability to make a new retromuscular pocket or the presence of visibly calcified capsules [9] or sick capsules (intense inflammatory process) would contraindicate the technique of making the new pectoral pocket.

In relation to other techniques, simple capsulorrhaphy, which consists of suturing between the anterior and posterior edges of the medial.

medial capsule, is not recommended due to high recurrence [19, 20]. Lateral or upper capsulectomy was not indicated in the reported cases, since with the change of plan, there was no healing restriction for the placement of implants. Bostwick suggests the correction of symmastia with excision of the central capsule and capsulorrhaphy of the flaps of the central capsules, associated with partial capsulectomies/lateral capsulotomies, in addition to textured implants for better adherence. Zingaretti et al. [21] describe a complex technique involving capsulectomy in the medial quadrant, adhesion points and medial capsulorrhaphy through transcutaneous points on the entire edge of the breast, but without changing the plan for placing the implants, which are necessarily smaller in order not to tension capsulorrhaphy points. Out of 10 retromuscular cases, it discriminates only 1 case after breast reconstruction.

Among the changes to a new pocket, the change from the submuscular plane to the subcutaneous plane, although suggested by some authors [8, 11] can be a less interesting option in many cases of primary cosmetic augmentation surgery, due to the possibility of palpation of the implant, capsular contracture or rippling development [16]. This would happen much more likely in cases of breast reconstruction. In addition, as in cases 2 and 3, it is possible to associate fat grafting in the same surgical procedure (for refinement of breast reconstruction). The option using acellular dermal matrices (ADM) to cover implants in the subcutaneous tissue would be an excellent option, but the cost is actually much higher, sometimes contraindicating the procedure. The change from the submammary to submuscular plane in cases of pre-pectoral symmastia is also widely performed [6].

Among the associated techniques, the use of dermal matrices facilitates and increases the possibility of correcting implant misplacement, in addition to integrating the matrix with the tissue [12]. However, the costs are high. Spear et al. [22], reported good results in their series of cases with the use of ADM used in breast reconstruction reviews: 5 cases of symmastia that were corrected with capsulorrhaphy with dermal graft medially (graft "onlay") or associated with confection change in the neo pectoral pocket, to avoid changing the implant to the old plan. Similarly, other authors also use a medial sling of the ROM to correct symmastia in cases of breast reconstruction [12, 23, 24] or cosmetic mammoplasty [25].

Parsa et al. [9] suggest anterior and posterior capsulectomy in the central region for its obliteration, and confection of a limited posterior capsule flap, followed by anterior capsulorrhaphy to make a new mammary board. This technique also depends on a posterior mature capsule (this dissection is already technically more difficult [9] in cases of retromuscular implants) and could also be used in retromammary stores. Foustanos and Zavrides [19] in only one case described capsulotomy and medial caspulorrhaphy associated with transcutaneous points to define the medial edges of the breasts.

The option for microtextured silicone prostheses was indicated, in principle, due to greater adherence [1] in relation to smooth implants (nanotexture). However, as a new pocket is made, these prostheses can also be used. Polyurethane prostheses could be used, especially in cases of subglandular or subfascial revision, since they do not undergo rotation or displacement, can improve rippling and capsular contracture [18]. Castello et al. [18] indicate polyurethane prostheses in the neosubpectoral pocket only in refractory cases of contracture.

As for the postoperative period, Kalaria et al. suggest that the patient rest between 4 and 6 weeks for abduction and lateral rotation of the humerus [11] due to the repositioning of the pectoralis major muscle. However, if the correction is adequate as suggested in the reports, such prolonged rest can be debilitating [7]. Therefore, conventional postoperative rest and the use of a bra with medial support in the adhesion area for 3 months were indicated to stabilize the surgical correction [2].

The only meta-analysis found [2] in relation to symmastia, although it does not reach conclusions about which surgical techniques are more efficient to correct it, describes an algorithm for both congenital and acquired symmastia. It advises the evaluation of the capsule as a more effective surgical procedure and, eventually, the combination with a muscle repair (which was done in this series of cases). The use of ADM would be reserved in cases of recurrence or for patients who desire large volume implants. The metaanalysis concludes by advising an integration of techniques to bring better results, as described in this article.

Finally, to avoid the occurrence of symmastia, Sanchez et al. [10] advise that when the access is inframammary, in addition to careful medial dissection, to start the elevation of the pectoralis major muscle medially and proceed laterally, with direct muscular visualization so that there is no elevation of the pectoralis minor muscle, since its fibers may be close to or intertwined with the costal insertion of the pectoralis major. The choice of the size/base of the implants in relation to the patient's chest is also essential, following directions from Selvaggi et al. [15] and Tebbetts [26].

7. Conclusion

Here we describe an integration of techniques for correction of retromuscular symmastia resulting from bilateral breast reconstruction with implants, namely, points of adhesion in the pre-sternal region and alteration of the breast implant pocket with anterior capsule flap, maintaining subpectoral space. The technique is easily reproducible and versatile, and can be used to correct other misplaced breast prostheses, as well as to correct capsular contractures. Furthermore, it can be associated with lipotransfer, usually beneficial for esthetic refinement in cases of breast reconstruction.

There were no displacements of the implants in the postoperative period or capsular contractures so far, and the patients reported being satisfied.

Author details

Márcia Balbina Lorenzo Hoyos
Rede de Assistência à Saúde Metropolitana, Sarandi-Paraná, Brazil

*Address all correspondence to: mblhoyos@gmail.com

IntechOpen

© 2023 The Author(s). Licensee IntechOpen. This chapter is distributed under the terms of the Creative Commons Attribution License (http://creativecommons.org/licenses/by/3.0), which permits unrestricted use, distribution, and reproduction in any medium, provided the original work is properly cited. (cc) BY

References

[1] Bostwick J III. Breast. St. Louis: Quality Medical Publishing; 2000

[2] Guillier D, Sapino G, Watfa W, Raffoul W, di Summa PG. Surgical treatment of symmastia: A systematic review of techniques, outcomes and complications. Journal of Plastic, Reconstructive & Aesthetic Surgery. 2020;**74**(3):P449-P462

[3] Spence RJ, Feldman JJ, Ryan JJ. Symmastia: The problem of medial confluence of the breasts. Plastic and Reconstructive Surgery. 1984;**73**(2):261-266. DOI: 10.1097/00006534-198402000-00020

[4] Spear SL, Little JW. Breast capsulorrhaphy. Plastic and Reconstructive Surgery. 1988;**81**(2):274-279. DOI: 10.1097/00006534-198802000-00026

[5] Parsa FD, Koehler SD, Parsa AA, Murariu D, Daher P. Symmastia after breast augmentation. Plastic and Reconstructive Surgery. 2011;**127**:63e-65e

[6] Khan UD. Correction of acquired synmastia with muscle-splitting biplane implant replacement. Aesthetic Plastic Surgery. 2009;**33**:605-610

[7] Hammond DC. Commentary on: Iatrogenic symmastia: Causes and suggested repair technique. Aesthetic Surgery Journal. 2019;**39**:873-874

[8] Lesavoy MA, Trussler AP, Dickinson BP. Difficulties with subpectoral augmentation mammaplasty and its correction: The role of subglandular site change in revision aesthetic breast surgery. Plastic and Reconstructive Surgery. 2010;**125**:363-371

[9] Parsa FD, Parsa AA, Koehler SM, Daniel M. Surgical correction of symmastia. Plastic and Reconstructive Surgery. 2010;**125**:1577-1579

[10] Sanchez ER, Sanchez R, Moliver C. Anatomic relationship of the pectoralis major and minor muscles: A cadaveric study. Aesthetic Surgery Journal. 2014;**34**:258-263

[11] Kalaria SS, Henderson J, Moliver CL. Iatrogenic symmastia: Causes and suggested repair technique. Aesthetic Surgery Journal. 2019;**39**:863-872

[12] Grabov-Nardini G, HaikJ RE, Winkler E. AlloDerm sling for correction of Synmastia after immediate, tissue expander, breast reconstruction in thin women. Eplasty. 2009;**9**:e54

[13] Pavelecini M, Fasolin FB, Zanin EM, Gasperin BDM, de Freitas Neto FM, Possamai LM, et al. Simastia pós-mamoplastia de aumento com implantes de silicone: Tratamento com suturas de adesão/post-mammoplasty symmastia augmentation with silicone implants: Treatment with quilting sutures. Revista Brasileira de Cirurgia Plástica. 2018;**33**(2):251-257

[14] Becker H, Shaw KE, Kara M. Correction of symmastia using an adjustable implant. Plastic and Reconstructive Surgery. 2005;**115**:21246

[15] Selvaggi G, Giordano S, Ishak L. Synmastia: Prevention and correction. Annals of Plastic Surgery. 2010;**65**:455-461

[16] Spear SL, Dayan JH, Bogue D, et al. The "neosubpectoral" pocket for the correction of symmastia. Plastic

and Reconstructive Surgery. 2009;**124**:695-703

[17] Maxwell GP, Birchenough SA, Gabriel A. Efficacy of neopectoral pocket in revisionary breast surgery. Aesthetic Surgery Journal. 2009;**29**:379-385

[18] Castello MF, Lazzeri D, Silvestri A, et al. Maximizing the use of precapsular space and the choice of implant type in breast augmentation mammaplasty revisions: Review of 49 consecutive procedures and patient satisfaction assessment. Aesthetic Plastic Surgery. 2011;**35**:828-838

[19] Foustanos A, Zavrides H. Surgical reconstruction of iatrogenic symmastia. Plastic and Reconstructive Surgery. 2008;**121**(3):143e-144e

[20] Yoo G, Lee PK. Capsular flaps for the management of malpositioned implants after augmentation mammoplasty. Aesthetic Surgery Journal. 2010;**34**(1):111-115

[21] Zingaretti N, De Biasio F, De Lorenzi F, Massarut S, Parodi PC. An efficient method for the correction of iatrogenic symmastia: A case series. Annals of Medicine and Surgery (London). 2018;**29**:14-18

[22] Spear SL, Sher SR, Al-Attar A, Pittman T. Applications of acellular dermal matrix in revision breast reconstruction surgery. Plastic and Reconstructive Surgery. 2014;**133**:1-10

[23] Nahabedian MY, Spear S. L, Acellular dermal matrix for secondary procedures following prosthetic breast reconstruction. Aesthetic Surgery Journal. 2011;**31**(7_Supplement):38S-50S

[24] Kaufman D. Pocket reinforcement using acellular dermal matrices in revisionary breast augmentation. Clinics in Plastic Surgery April. 2012;**39**(2):137-148

[25] Baxter RA. Intracapsular allogenic dermal grafts for breast implant-related problems. Plastic and Reconstructive Surgery. 2003;**112**:16926; discussion 7-8

[26] Tebbetts JB, Adams WP. Five critical decisions in breast augmentation using five measurements in 5 minutes: The high five decision support process. Plastic and Reconstructive Surgery. 2005;**116**:2005-2016

Chapter 12

Revisions for Complications of Aesthetic Breast Surgery

Angelo Cuzalina, Pasquale G. Tolomeo and Victoria A. Mañón

Abstract

Breast surgery continues to be one of the most sought-after cosmetic procedures in recent years. Patients are opting to undergo various procedures to enhance the aesthetics and appearance of their breasts. The goal of any cosmetic procedure is to compliment one's body and achieve satisfactory results. However, some patients may experience complications or become dissatisfied with the final result. These complications include breast asymmetry, implant malposition, implant deflation, rippling, and capsular contracture. Aesthetic breast revision is a highly specialized procedure that requires an experienced surgeon, aiming to address the patient's concerns as well as achieve a more desirable outcome.

Keywords: aesthetic breast surgery, breast revision, implant malposition, capsular contraction, breast mastopexy, breast augmentation

1. Introduction

Breast surgery is one of the most sought-after cosmetic treatments with breast augmentation being the most common aesthetic procedure [1]. Patients may undergo various procedures to enhance and improve the appearance of their breasts. Breast surgery can be divided into breast augmentation with the use of implants or autologous fat transfer, mastopexy, reduction mammaplasty, or a combination of these procedures. The aesthetic outcomes rely on postoperative breast symmetry, size, and shape. Beauty is in the eye of the beholder, and it is greatly influenced by an individual's perception, as well as symmetrical balance. Aesthetic breast surgery is the congruence of science and art based on the relationship between human morphology and anthropometric proportions.

As with any procedure, there are associated risks with breast surgery including asymmetry, rippling, implant malposition, implant deflation, or capsular contracture. The goal of aesthetic revisional breast surgery is to address the unsatisfactory result or complication of the previous breast surgery and produce an aesthetic result. The benefits of revisional breast surgery are numerous. Patients can achieve a more desirable breast size and shape, correct any complications from previous breast surgery, and improve their self-confidence and body image.

However, revision breast surgery is not without risks. The surgery carries the same risks as other surgical procedures such as bleeding, infection, and anesthesia complications. The risks of revision surgery are greater than the risks of the initial breast surgery due to the presence of scar tissue, altered anatomy, and compromized blood supply, increasing the risk of tissue/nipple necrosis.

Aesthetic revision breast surgery is a complex procedure that requires a skilled and experienced surgeon to achieve optimal results. Patients should carefully research potential surgeons and choose a surgeon who has extensive experience performing breast revision surgery.

The surgical aspect of breast surgery continues to evolve over time with advancements in surgical techniques and a greater knowledge of anatomy and its variants. The surgeon must have an armamentarium of surgical techniques to offer treatment that promises both aesthetic results and longevity with marginal risk of complications. As the technical aspect of surgery improves, knowledge of the anatomy is the single aspect of breast surgery that remains consistent. Being equipped with this knowledge allows the surgeon to identify and preserve important structures, therefore decreasing the risk of complications and improving the final outcome.

2. Preoperative planning

The preoperative patient appointment is one of the most important steps in the breast revision process. Most patients seek evaluations from multiple surgeons, and it is crucial to make a great impression. The goal of the consult is to determine the patient's surgical goals, obtain medical information, perform a physical exam, develop a diagnosis, explain the recommended procedures with associated risks and benefits, and address the patient's expectations. It is the appointment where patients should be properly educated about the condition(s) and procedure options while establishing realistic expectations.

2.1 Patient evaluation

Preoperative evaluation of a patient is vital to any surgical procedure. First and foremost, it is imperative to review the patient's medical history and chief complaint. The chief complaint is the primary topic of discussion and must be in the patient's own words. The patient should be able to describe their concerns and may be guided with open-ended questions. A thorough evaluation should include medical diagnoses, medications with proper dosages and frequencies, allergies, and past surgical history. The patient's social history must be obtained, and the discussion must focus on the use of tobacco or nicotine-containing products due to concerns of compromised vasculature and wound healing. Finally, social history should include the patient's profession as the patient may have restrictions of their work-related duties. Lastly, the surgeon should determine if there is any family history of cancer, as well as any previous mammograms. Those patients over the age of 40 or patients who are of high risk should undergo a mammography prior to surgery [2].

2.2 Patient examination

The physical examination begins with a visual inspection of the breasts. The key areas to evaluate during the breast examination are the skin envelope (laxity and quality), breast volume, position of the nipple-areola complex, areolar size, degree of ptosis, asymmetries, and pocket location of the implants. Mallucci and Branford stated the four pivotal elements in breast aesthetics are: proportion of the upper pole to lower pole, angulation of the nipple, upper pole slope, and lower pole convexity [3].

The surgeon must be able to identify any asymmetries, implant malposition, and size discrepancies. It is important to note that a size difference of <10% is considered within normal limits [4]. Aside from breast morphology, the surgeon must also identify any deformities of the chest or spine that may lead to an asymmetry. Lastly, the breasts and axilla should be palpated to evaluate for the presence of masses or lymphadenopathy, including the associated lymphatic chain of the supraclavicular and axillary lymph nodes.

A grading system to evaluate breast ptosis was developed by Dr. Paule Regnault. The grade of breast ptosis is determined by the position of the nipple in relation to the inframammary fold (IMF) and skin envelope (**Figure 1**, **Table 1**) [5].

The last part of the examination involves obtaining breast measurements and photos (**Figure 2**). These measurements include: [3, 4, 6–8].

1. Breast width (BW): Measurement of the most medial to the anterior axillary line
2. Breast thickness (BT): Measurement of the thickness of the upper pole
3. Sternal notch to nipple (SN-N): Ideal measurement of 19–21 cm
4. Mid-clavicle to areola (MC-A): ideal measurement of 19–21 cm
5. Inter-nipple distance: Ideal measurement of 19–21 cm

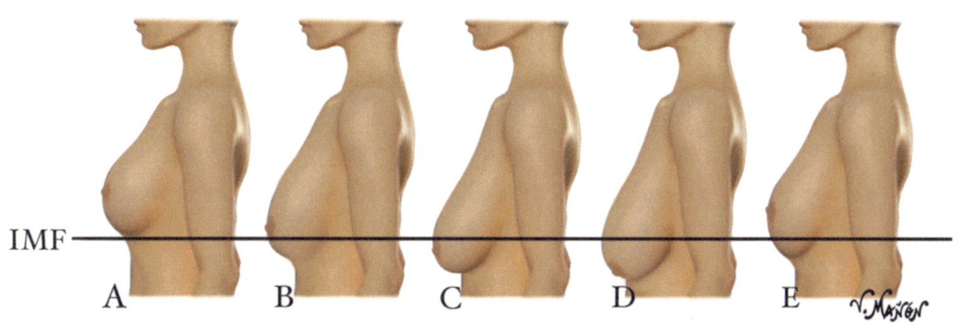

Figure 1.
Breast ptosis classification [5]. A: normal, B: 1st degree, C: 2nd degree, D: 3rd degree, and E: glandular ptosis.

Regnault's classification of ptosis	
Minor ptosis (1st degree)	Nipple at the IMF or 1 cm inferior to IMF
Moderate ptosis (2nd degree)	Nipple inferior to IMF & superior to lower breast contour
Severe ptosis (3rd degree)	Nipple inferior to IMF & at lower breast contour
Glandular ptosis	Nipple superior to IMF & breast tissue inferior to the breast fold
Pseudoptosis	Nipple superior to IMF; breast is hypoplastic and inferior to the breast fold

Table 1.
Regnault's classification of breast ptosis [5].

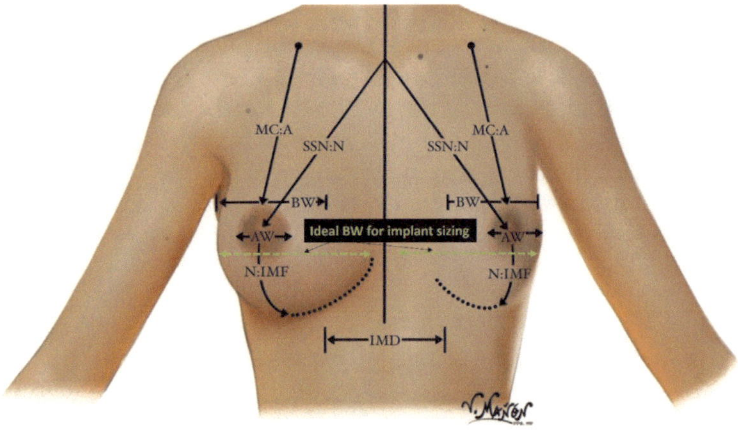

Figure 2.
Breast measurements and 'ideal' base width.

6. Areolar width (AW): Ideal measurement of 3.5–4.5 cm

7. Nipple to inframammary fold (N-IMF): Ideal measurement of 7–8 cm

8. Intermammary distance (IMD): Ideal measurement of 21 cm from nipple to nipple

9. Ptosis: Nipple position in reference to inframammary fold

10. Mid-humeral point (MHP): Mid-point between the acromion and lateral epicondyle and the ideal location of the nipple

11. Breast parenchyma size: Lower pole is greater than the upper pole.

12. Skin quality

13. Parenchyma quality and elasticity

The most crucial measurements in breast revision surgery are the breast width, sternal notch to nipple, and nipple to inframammary fold. The 'ideal' or desired base width (BW) is typically different from the actual BW of the native breast tissue and can most often be measured as the distance from the anterior axillary line to within 1 cm from the chest midline. The goal or desired base width for the patient is used during implant sizing to achieve the ideal implant width (**Figure 2**). The breast width measurement assesses for the maximal implant width to avoid symmastia or lateral position of the breast implant. The nipple to inframammary fold measurement is critical to establish an esthetic lower pole fullness and overall breast shape. The sternal notch to nipple measurement determines the location of the nipple-areolar complex on the chest wall [6]. The surgeon must acknowledge these measurements and respect the limitations of the breast tissue.

The preoperative evaluation is imperative in order to allow for the surgeon to develop a sound surgical approach to achieve the best aesthetic outcome.

2.3 Patient discussion

The patient and the surgeon must be aware that no breasts are similar in shape and size and furthermore, breasts are rarely perfectly symmetrical. The surgeon must address the patient's desires while maintaining sound surgical parameters. The patient should be an active participant in the consultation by providing the chief complaint and expressing the desired outcomes. A well-educated patient understands the indications for various procedures and is aware of any limitations or possible complications. This assures a great provider patient experience with an aesthetic outcome.

3. Surgical complications

3.1 Implant malposition

Breast asymmetry is a common phenomenon in which there is a difference in shape, size, and/or position between each breast. One of the most common causes of asymmetry is implant malposition.

Implant malposition can occur due to improper implant selection, inadequate tissue support, or surgical error. The implant may shift in a superior, medial, inferior, or lateral direction. Shifting may be due to an inadequate or excessive pocket size, as well as poor tissue architecture.

Superior displacement is due to inadequate release of the inferior aspect of the breast pocket, causing the implant to slide upwards. Medial displacement creates symmastia (confluence of the breasts) due to excessive medial dissection of the breast pocket. Over dissection of the inferior aspect of the breast, poor tissue support, or large implants may lead to inferior displacement of the implant, resulting in thinning of the breast tissue and skin, as well as ptosis.

Lateral malposition is one of the most common types, where the implant is positioned along the armpits, creating a wide gap between the breasts. Over time, these implants may cause pain or tenderness and may be palpable and visible. Additional causes of implant malposition include trauma, capsular contraction, or aberrant anatomy.

To minimize the development of implant malposition, the surgeon must be thorough with the initial surgical planning. The surgeon must focus on selecting the proper implant that does not violate the natural breast width, complementing the patient's body, and avoiding over/under dissection of the breast pocket. Postoperatively, patients must adhere to minimizing strenuous activities for several weeks to avoid disruption of the breast pocket, as well as utilizing compression garments to maintain the position of the implants.

3.2 Capsular contracture

Following breast augmentation, the body develops a capsule or scar tissue around the implant. A healthy breast capsule is soft and assists with maintaining the breast implant in its position. Capsular contracture develops when the body's immune system has an increased sensitivity to the implant or is activated in response to the presence of a bacterial biofilm or blood, producing a thickened and tightened breast capsule. This may lead to distortion of the breast shape, hardening of the breast, pain, and tenderness.

The exact mechanism of capsular contracture is unknown. However, steps may be taken to reduce the incidence of capsular contracture. Surgically, the surgeon must adhere to proper sterile techniques and minimize direct handling of the implant. The breast pocket must be free of any active bleeding, as well as residual blood. The implant should be washed with sterile saline and a triple antibiotic solution to reduce the formation of a biofilm. Patients are instructed to avoid direct contact with the breasts and adhere to postoperative instructions. Prophylactic montelukast or zafirlukast has shown to reduce the incidence of capsular contracture by reducing inflammation around the implant [9]. The incidence of capsular contracture cases requiring revision surgery is 10% at 10 years, with a decrease prevalence in implants placed in a submuscular plane [10].

3.3 Implant rippling/deflation

Implant rippling is due to the folding of the edges of the implant creating a visible wrinkle along the skin. Implant rippling occurs more often in patients with thin breast tissue (minimal tissue coverage), as well as inadequately filled implants (edges of the implant will fold over itself).

Implant deflation may be caused by a rupture or leak leading to the loss of the implants size and shape. Immediate deflation is more common with saline implants creating a drastic change in the breast appearance, while rupture of silicone implants may not cause any changes. Potential causes of implant deflation are a manufacturing defect, trauma, or weakening of the implant capsule.

Prevention of implant rippling/deflation focuses on selecting an appropriate implant size, cohesiveness, and pocket position to allow for adequate soft tissue coverage.

4. Breast revision

Upon completion of the patient examination, the surgeon must determine what is the best procedure to address the patient's concerns and rectify the complication.

4.1 Post-augmentation breast ptosis

Following augmentation, a "waterfall effect" may form due to the sliding of breast tissue (ptosis) over the fixed implant [11]. Options for correction of ptosis include implant exchange, removal of implants, mastopexy, or no treatment.

If the patient is happy with the position, shape, and cleavage of the breasts, no surgical intervention is required.

For patients who are unhappy with the shape and position of the breasts, a decision is to be made whether to place a larger implant or shift the implant pocket to a sub-glandular position. The surgeon must be mindful that if lower pole ptosis is present, switching to a sub-glandular position will cause the 'waterfall effect' to persist.

The most definitive treatment to address the "waterfall effect" is a mastopexy. The breast mastopexy aims to recreate a symmetrical, appropriately sized breast while reducing breast ptosis [6]. The procedure involves elevating the nipple-areolar complex (NAC) in addition to removing excess skin and breast tissue. The mastopexy incision depends on the degree of ptosis and desired outcome (**Table 2**).

Mastopexy incision design	Indications	Advantages	Disadvantages
Periareolar/ crescent	Grade I or II ptosis and nipple asymmetry	1. NAC elevation 1–2 cm 2. Camouflaged scar	1. Decreased projection of breast mound 2. Scar Widening
Vertical/ teardrop	All ptosis grades	1. Correction of ptosis and resection of excess tissue 2. Preservation of nipple mound projection	1. Possible persistent asymmetry 2. Decreased lower pole projection
Wise pattern/ inverted T	Grade II or III ptosis	1. Increased resection of breast parenchyma and skin 2. Allows for breast reduction and lift in conjunction with augmentation	1. Increased scar presence 2. Increased suture spitting

Table 2.
Mastopexy design [12].

4.1.1 Periareolar/crescent

The periareolar technique may be utilized in patients who with Grade I/II ptosis or nipple asymmetry and mild skin excess. This technique allows the surgeon to elevate the nipple-areolar complex within 2 cm, with minimal reduction of redundant tissue or skin. This procedure assists with balancing out the nipples with minimal effect on the breast parenchyma. In regard to reduction of the skin envelope, a periareolar defect may develop and lead to poor wound healing, distortion of the NAC, and decreased breast projection [6].

The downside of this procedure is the postoperative periareolar widening. Two methods may be utilized to reduce this risk. First, maximal stretch should be applied while creating the incision to minimize the effects of the immediate postoperative stretching. Second, the use of a permanent purse-string suture for closure of the incision. This allows for stress absorption by the suture and reduction in tension along the areola. The most common suture used is a polytetrafluoroethylene (PTFE) suture [6].

The crescent mastopexy is a modified version of the periareolar technique that includes resection of circumareolar breast tissue. The crescent incision may be utilized in patients with an asymmetrical nipple or those requiring NAC elevation of 1–2 cm.

Benelli discussed a periareolar mastopexy that incorporates parenchymal restructuring [13]. This procedure allows the surgeon to reduce larger breasts while utilizing the periareolar approach. The inferior breast parenchyma is excised vertically, and the parenchymal pillars are repositioned to reduce the fullness of the lower pole while simultaneously elevating the breast position.

Based on the authors' belief and the literature, periareolar mastopexies have an increased rate of revision due to undesirable results such as poor esthetics, inadequate projection, and high recurrence rates [12, 14].

4.1.2 Vertical-teardrop

The vertical mastopexy focuses on repositioning the NAC and correcting breast ptosis by allowing for excision of glandular tissue, ultimately improving the longevity of the procedure. This mastopexy involves a periareolar incision with a vertical component.

The Hall-Findlay technique is frequently used due to the versatility in pedicle design, minimal scar presence, and improved projection. This technique is supported by a superior-medial-central (SMC) or a medio-central (MC) pedicle due to its robust arterial supply and venous drainage. A wedge resection of the inferior pole breast parenchyma is performed, while the remaining medial and lateral pillars are re-approximated to provide support to the NAC, ultimately reducing the breast volume and elevating the breast [15]. Of note, the inferior aspect of the vertical incision must be placed superior to the inframammary fold (IMF) to avoid an incision along the abdomen; this is due to the tendency of the IMF to elevate with time.

For implant pocket selection, a sub-glandular or sub-pectoralis implant placement is both viable options, this is due to the preservation of the 2nd/3rd internal mammary perforators [12]. With this technique, the breast will have moderate upper pole fullness with a compressed inferior pole. It will take several months for the implant to settle and the inferior pole to develop its shape.

4.1.3 Wise pattern/inverted T

The Wise Pattern/Inverted T is one of the most versatile mastopexy techniques allowing for a large reduction of both breast parenchyma and skin with simultaneous implant placement. This technique allows for a multitude of pedicle options, including inferior, superior, medial, central pedicles, or a combination [14]. This mastopexy consists of two components: the vertical and horizontal incisions. The vertical incision allows for elevation of the NAC, as well as reduction of the inferior pole. The horizontal incision allows for excision of ptotic skin/breast parenchyma while controlling the nipple to inframammary fold distance; this ensures an aesthetic lower pole shape.

The surgeon must be aware of the limitations of this technique. If an inferior pedicle is utilized, there is an increased incidence of redundant inferior breast pole or bottoming out of the implant due to a reduced pillar of support along the inferior pole [16]. An additional concern is the significant scarring compared to the previously discussed techniques. When performing a combined mastopexy and augmentation, there is an increased incidence of tissue dehiscence along the trifurcation due to the weight of the overlying implant [12].

4.1.4 Surgeon's preference

With revision surgery, the surgeon must develop a definitive plan and inform the patient of potential complications. All prior operative reports should be obtained to determine the original planes of dissection and selected pedicle design, reducing the risk of further complications. In cases where the pedicle design is unknown, a pedicle design with multiple perforators is ideal. The superomedial-central (SMC) is the surgeon's preferred pedicle for SN-N distances less than 30 cm due to the robust blood supply both medially and centrally (**Figure 3**).

The surgeon must be aware of various pedicle designs and their appropriate applications (**Figure 4**). The superior-medial pedicle (SM), when combined with a central pedicle (C), is the most versatile pedicle due to its robust blood supply. The pedicle is perfused by the internal mammary artery in addition to the 2nd-4th internal mammary perforators (superior-medial-pedicle) and the trans-pectoral perforators off the internal mammary and medial mammary branches (central pedicle). The minimal

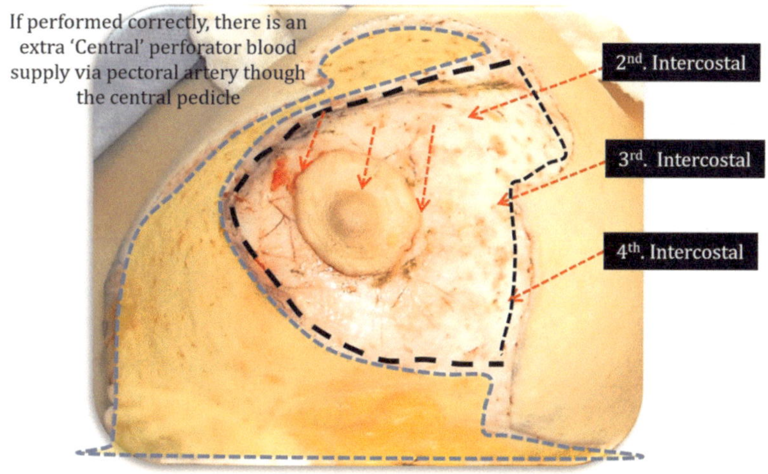

Figure 3.
Superomedial-central pedicle. This pedicle design demonstrates the excellent dual blood supply to the breast and NAC via *medial, as well as central perforators.*

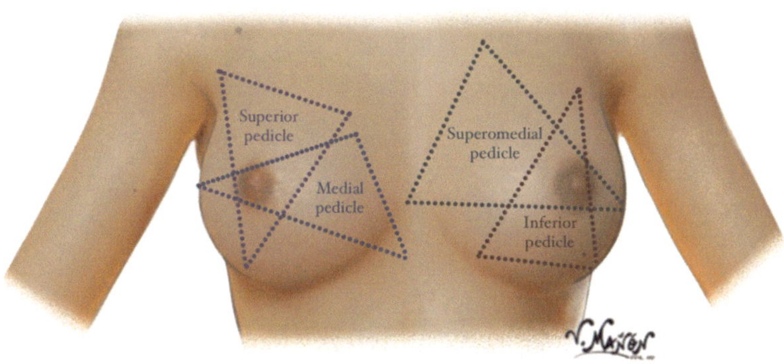

Figure 4.
Breast pedicles. The pedicle designs demonstrate the robust blood supply to the breast and NAC.

base width of the pedicle is 6–10 cm, ensuring adequate perfusion. If the patient has undergone previous augmentation with placement of the implant in a sub-glandular plane, the blood supply of the central pedicle is no longer viable (**Figure 5**).

The authors may select to utilize a different pedicle design depending on the surgical circumstance. For those patients with severe ptosis/pendulous breasts (SN-N > 30 cm), a medio-central (MC) pedicle allows the pedicle to rotate superiorly while preserving the vasculature and minimizing tension. The medio-central pedicle is perfused by the internal mammary artery and the arterial perforators (**Figure 6**) [17]. In cases of mild to moderate ptosis (NAC positioned 2–3 cm inferior to the IMF), a superior-medial-central (SMC) allows for improvement of upper pole fullness and shape. This pedicle is perfused by the lateral and internal mammary arteries, as well as a branch of the axillary artery; this robust blood supply reduces the risk of wound dehiscence [17].

In regard to implant pocket selection, the authors routinely select a total submuscular plane. The total submuscular plane preserves the blood supply to the

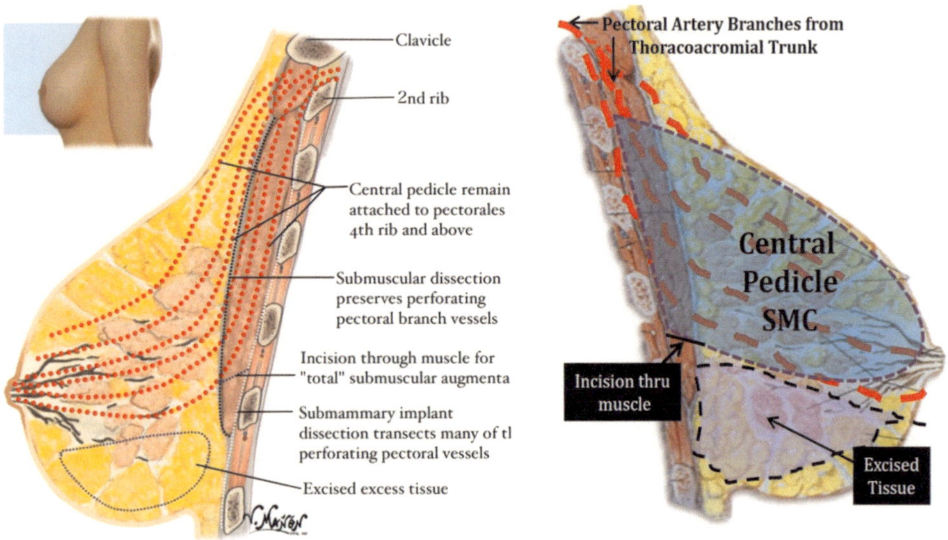

Figure 5.
Pectoral vessels. Sub-mammary pocket development disrupts the perforators to the central pedicle. A total submuscular implant placement preserves the perforating pectoral branches to the central portion of the pedicle even with major inferior gland excision.

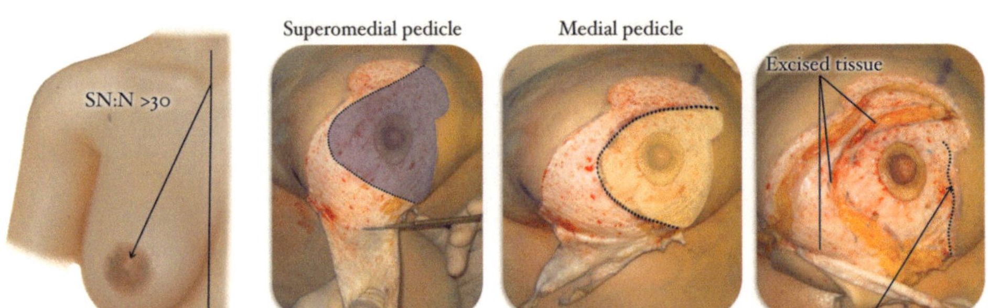

Figure 6.
The superomedial pedicle. The SMC pedicle is utilized for most mastopexy cases. For patients with a SN-N greater than 30 cm, a MC pedicle is preferred due to its ease of rotation of the NAC with minimal constriction.

overlying pedicle while providing a layer of protection over the implant. The additional soft tissue coverage decreases the incidence of capsular contracture. The surgeon must properly prepare the pocket and ensure adequate release of the muscle. Improper release of the pocket may lead to a superiorly positioned implant creating significant upper pole fullness with a downward rotation of the NAC [6]. Additional pocket development below the serratus anterior and external obliques allows for additional coverage along the lateral and inferior aspect of the implant, increasing the support around the implant (**Figures** 7 and **8**). The surgeon must avoid excess dissection along the medial, inferomedial, and inferior aspects to avoid symmastia, boxy appearance of the medial breast and inferior displacement of the implant, respectively [6].

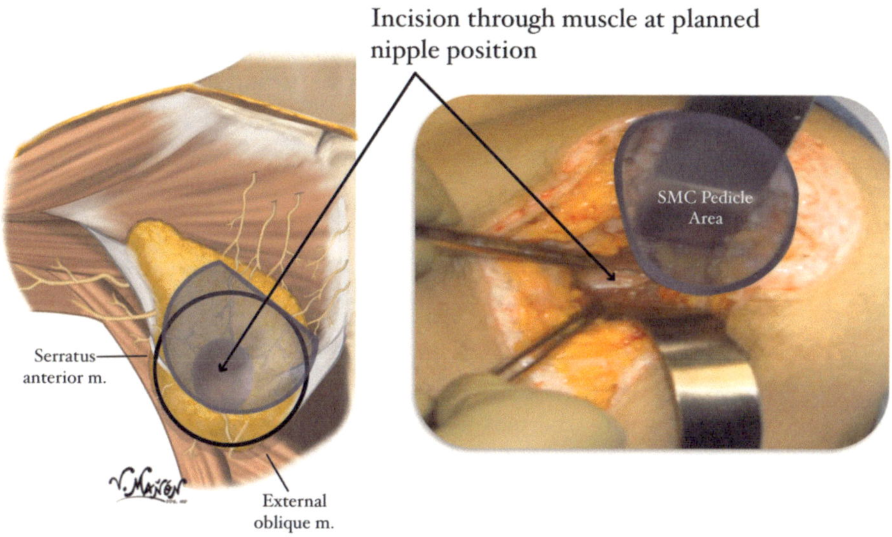

Figure 7.
The superomedial-central pedicle. The use of the SMC pedicle allows for the development of a total submuscular pocket. The submuscular pocket allows for complete coverage of the implant; this protects the implant as well as reduces the risk of bottoming out.

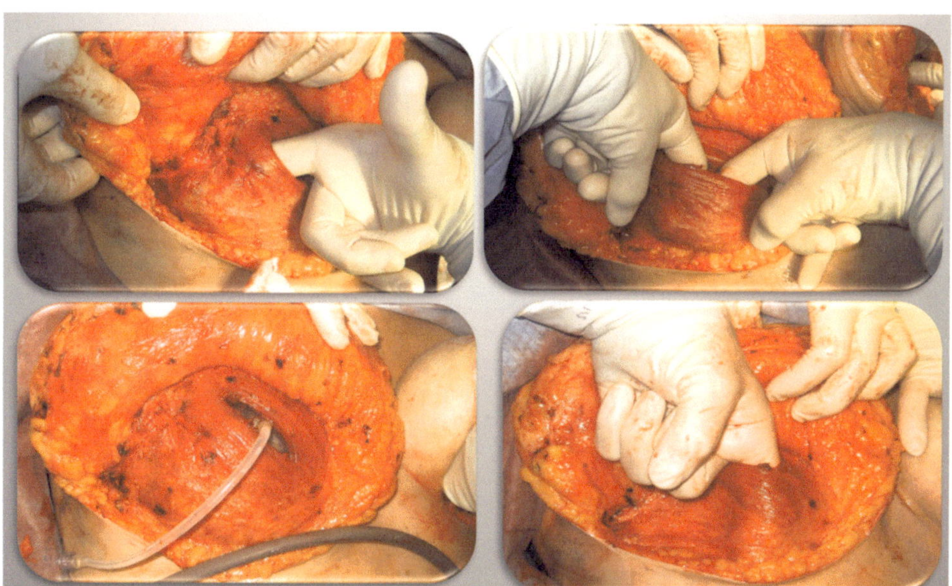

Figure 8.
Total submuscular pocket. Digital dissection allows for the development of a total submuscular flap. The surgeon must take caution during the dissection to avoid perforation of the flap, most specifically along the inferior aspect.

The most conservative approach to combined mastopexy and augmentation is for placement of the implant followed by the mastopexy. This permits for adequate parenchyma resection and skin removal. The authors proceed with the mastopexy followed by the augmentation. When performing the mastopexy first, the surgeon is able to create a total submuscular pocket and manipulate the breast tissue to improve the breast contours, as well as the implant projection. The skilled surgeon must properly plan the resection margin and select the appropriate implant in the preoperative appointment to avoid excess tissue/skin removal risking necrosis.

4.2 Implant malposition

Another complication is implant malposition, seen in both primary augmentation and combined augmentation/mastopexy. The implant is commonly displaced inferiorly and laterally can be addressed with pocket modifications, including capsulorraphies/capsulectomies.

Breast capsulorrhaphy, also known as an internal bra lift, is a surgical procedure, where the breast capsule is repaired and tightened. Capsulorraphy may be performed utilizing a multilayered suture, thermal energy, mesh, or a combination of these techniques. Spear discussed utilizing a multilayered suture with an absorbable or non-

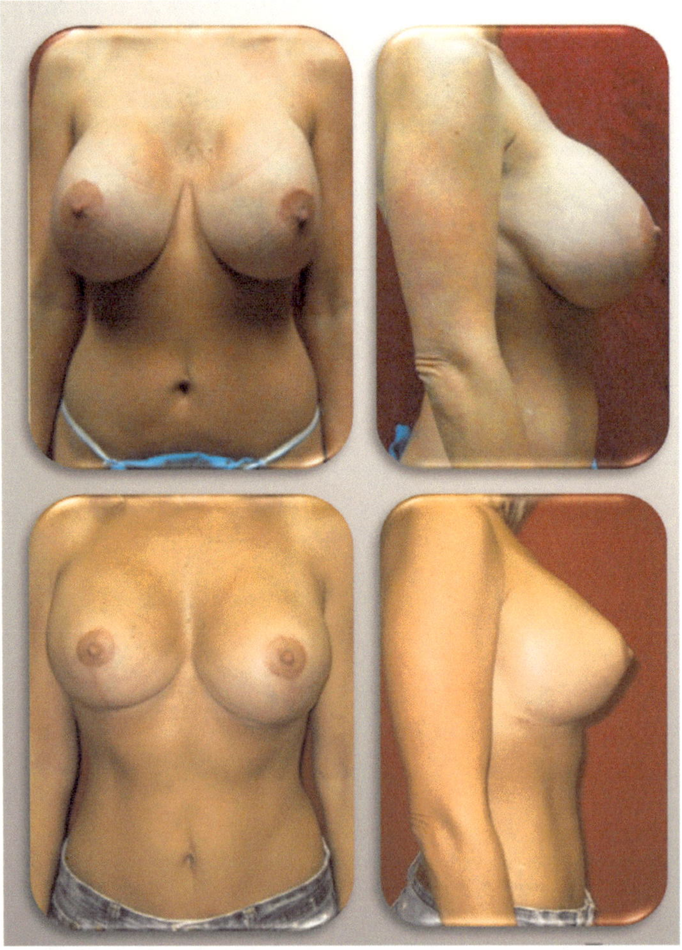

Figure 9.
Inferior displacement of the breast implants. The patient underwent previous breast augmentation and was unhappy with the "droopiness" of her breast tissue, as well as the position of the breast implants. The patient underwent a simultaneous lift and revision augmentation. A capsulorraphy was performed to reposition the breast higher on the chest wall.

resorbable suture allowing for correction in multiple increments and reducing stress on each individual suture [18]. "Popcorn" capsulorraphy was first described by Randquist. With this procedure, thermal energy is applied to the capsule, tightening and reshaping the pocket [19]. The Gala FLEX mesh scaffold is composed of resorbable poly-4-hydroxybutyrate monofilament fibers. The mesh provides an internal support along the breast capsule [20]. The scaffold allows for tissue ingrowth creating a vascularized tissue bed that integrates with the native tissue. The scaffold yields a final tissue strength three to five times stronger than native tissue, creating a more supported pocket [21].

For correction of the malposition implant, the authors utilize the multilayered suture technique into addition to the "popcorn" capsulorraphy. Preoperatively, the patient is evaluated in a standing position, and the proposed capsulorrpahy is performed and marked on the skin. It is also important to mark the areas of proposed capsulotomy to allow for re-positioning and decrease the pressure on the area of repair. Intraoperatively, an incision is made along the previous inframammary incision and the breast capsule is entered. The implant is removed and evaluated to ensure

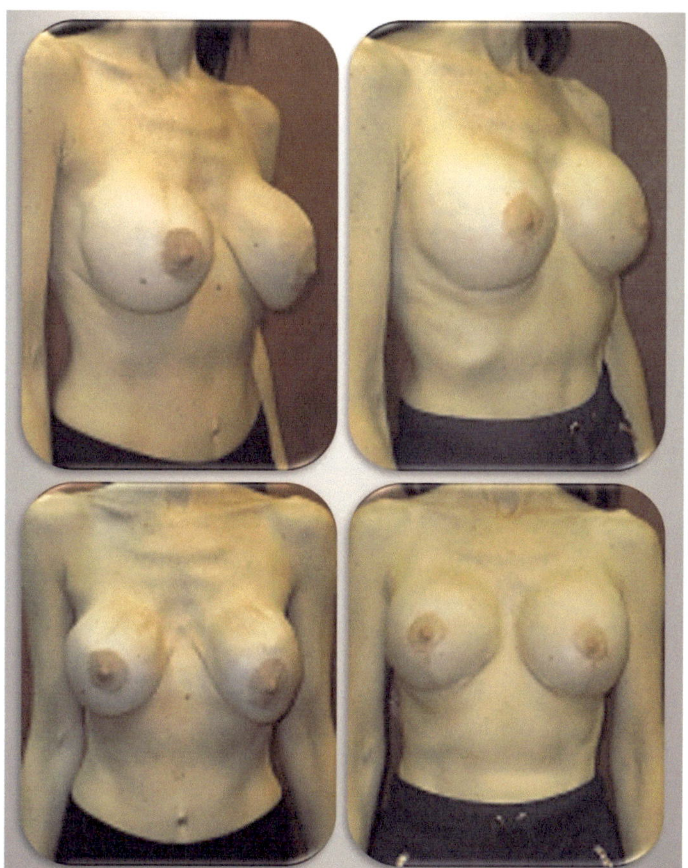

Figure 10.
Replacement above to below muscle. The patient shown is before and 3 months after switching implants from saline to silicone and changing her pocket from above muscle to a total submuscular position along with a simultaneous breast lift. The implants have a larger base width to further improve cleavage. The "total" submuscular placement produces improved implant coverage while also preventing slippage of the new implant into the old sub-mammary pocket.

that the implant is intact. Next, following the planned capsulorraphy, a Bovie cautery is utilized to score the capsule internally. This process creates a "popping" sound as the energy is applied to the breast capsule. Then, a suture capsulorraphy is performed along the treated area using a one Nurolon in a continuous-locking fashion. Once this is complete, mirroring capsulotomies are performed. The capsulotomies are performed opposite of the capsulorraphy, as well as along the anterior aspect of the capsule to allow for adequate repositioning. Upon completion of the capsulorraphy/ capsulotomy, the pocket is irrigated with triple antibiotic solution and betadine. The implant is re-inserted, the pocket is re-approximated, and the patient is placed in a beach chair position to confirm symmetry. Once symmetry is achieved, the patient is placed in the supine position, and the incision is closed in a layered fashion (**Figure 9**).

Some cases that have malpositioned implants above the muscle required removal and replacement into a near pocket below muscle. Some surgeons elect to use an ADM from the lateral border of pectoralis to prevent slippage of the implant back above muscle. However, the use of a total submuscular pocket in these cases prevents unwanted implant migration without the need for a costly ADM. The new total

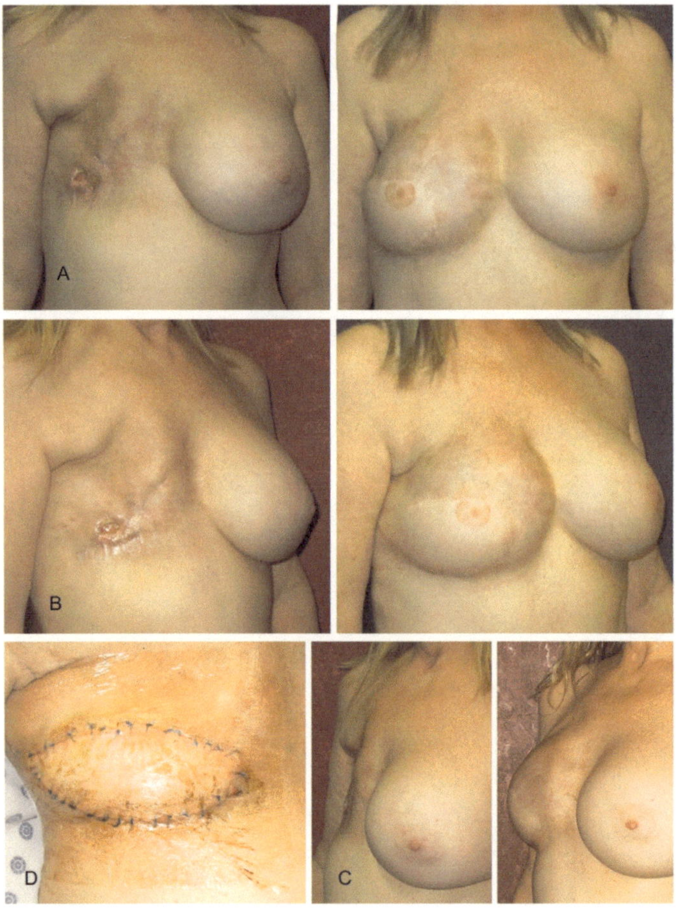

Figure 11.
Soft tissue reconstruction. Patient with previous mastectomy and radiation. Patient developed tissue necrosis with exposure of her rib. A latissimus dorsi flap (myocutaneous flap) was utilized to reconstruct the right breast tissue. Breast implant expanders were placed after surgery followed by final implants and nipple tattooing.

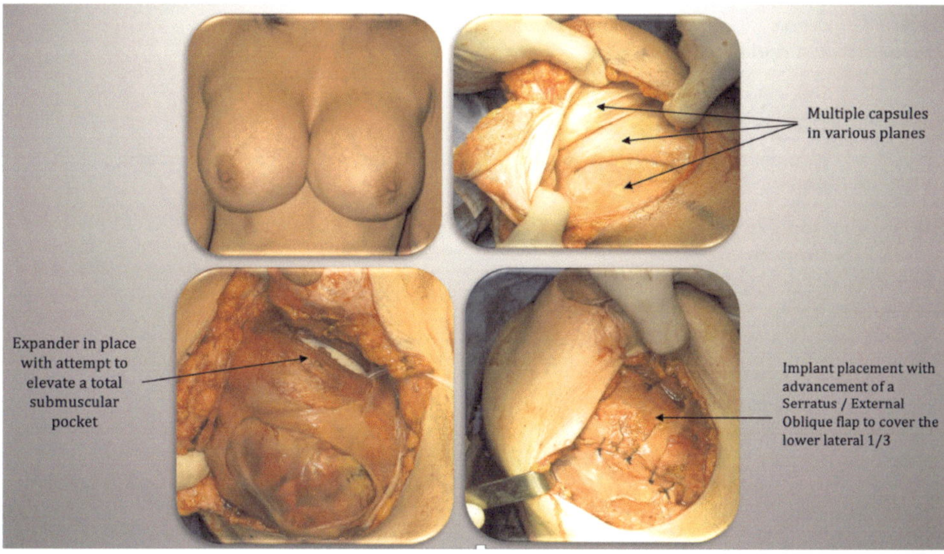

Figure 12.
Multiple breast revision surgeries. The above patient had undergone several breast augmentations with the final augmentation complicated by symmastia. The overlying muscle was significantly damaged and an inferolateral submuscular flap (serratus and external oblique muscles) was developed to obtain coverage over the new implant.

submuscular position is much easier to achieve when the patient requires a simultaneous mastopexy. The surgeon must use caution since the blood supply to the NAC has been compromized from their previous sub-mammary augmentation (**Figure 10**).

For difficult cases where there is a high risk of malposition recurrence, a mesh may be placed to reinforce the capsule. Prior to placement of the mesh, fascial flaps are prepared along the planned surgical area. The flaps will provide coverage over the mesh. The Gala FLEX mesh is placed along the weakened capsule or the area of a tissue deficit. Once properly positioned, the mesh is secured to the capsule and pectoralis muscle. Additional support may be provided by securing the mesh to the ribs. The authors utilize a 0 Vicryl in a continuous running fashion to secure the mesh to the underlying tissue, as well as ribs, recreating the internal support. Next, the mesh is fixated to the overlying fascial flap to provide additional soft tissue coverage using a 0 Vicryl.

For those patients with compromized soft tissue coverage, localized muscle flaps are a viable option for breast reconstruction to provide implant coverage and restore tissue defects (**Figures 11** and **12**).

4.3 Capsular contracture

Capsular contraction develops due to the excess scar formation around the breast implant causing hardening and distortion of the breast. Risk factors associated with the development of capsular contracture are a history of capsular contracture, subglandular implant placement, silicone rupture, smoking, bacterial contamination, and autoimmune disorders. Development of contracture is a continuous process that can present several years after implant placement [22].

Evaluation for capsular contracture is based on clinical exam. The provider must assess for any changes in the breast symmetry, texture, and appearance, as well as the patient's symptoms (**Table 3**). Additional modalities, ultrasound or magnetic

Baker grade	Breast description	Implant description	Treatment
I	Soft, normal shape	Non-palpable	No treatment
II	Firm, normal shape	Palpable, not visible	Nonsteroidal anti-inflammatory medications, Montelukast, capsulotomy
III	Firm, slight distortion	Palpable, visible	Capsulectomy, implant exchange
IV	Hard, severe distortion	Palpable, visible	Capsulectomy, implant exchange

Table 3.
Baker grade of capsular contracture [23].

resonance imaging (MRI), may be utilized to assess the extent of contracture and implant integrity.

Treatment of breast implant capsular contracture is based on the clinical presentation. In mild cases, the patient may be instructed to monitor for any progression of the capsular contracture, perform daily massages to soften the breast capsule, or take medications such as montelukast to reduce inflammation.

For moderate to severe cases (Grade III/IV), the surgeon must intervene to improve the patient's outcome. Surgical options include capsulotomy, capsulectomy,

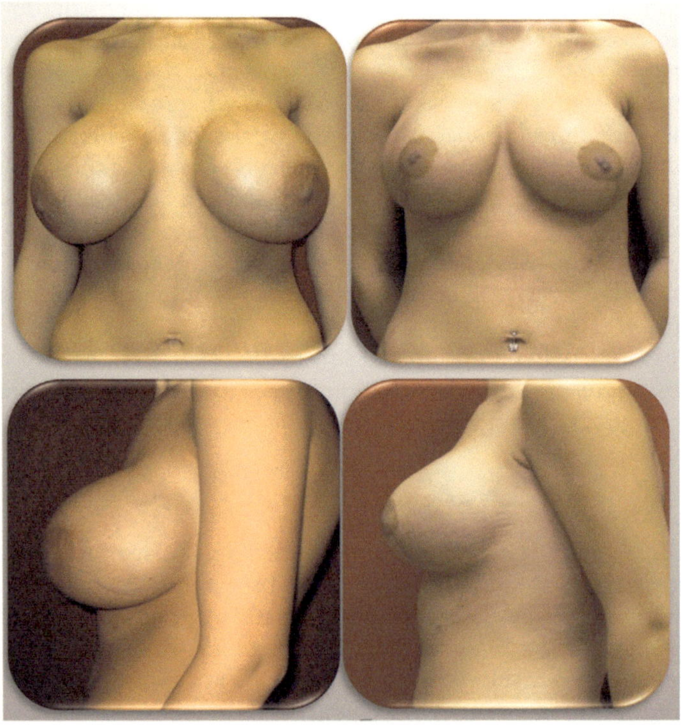

Figure 13.
Grade IV capsular contracture. Patient with grade IV capsular contracture. Patients with capsular contraction who desire a breast lift with augmentation must be informed of the high revision rate and risk of complications.

implant pocket change, use of acellular dermal matrices (ADM), or soft tissue/muscle flaps [24]. Studies demonstrate a success rate of 79% for reoperation with implant exchange. However, the recurrence rate is approximately 54% [25].

For correction of severe capsular contraction, the surgeon prefers to remove the capsule and implant en bloc to avoid silicone leakage into the breast cavity. The previous implant must be removed due to the concern for possible biofilm embedded along the implant shell. Once the affected capsule has been removed, the surgeon must determine the location of the previous implant pocket. If the implant was in a sub-glandular plane, a submuscular pocket will be developed to house the new implant. If a submuscular plane was utilized previously, the surgeon must determine the integrity of the remaining pectoralis pocket and whether an ADM or tissue flap must be utilized to recreate the breast pocket (**Figures 13** and **14**).

Acellular dermal matrix may provide a protection against capsular contracture. Studies demonstrate a decrease in blood vessel proliferation, fibroblast activity, fibrosis, and collagen deposition in addition to decreasing the inflammatory response of the body [26, 27].

Prior to placement of the mesh, soft tissue flaps are prepared along the planned surgical area. The flaps will provide coverage over the mesh. The Gala FLEX mesh is placed along the weakened capsule or the area of a tissue deficit. Once properly positioned, the mesh is secured to the underlying tissue and pectoralis muscle. Additional support may be provided by securing the mesh to the ribs. The authors utilize a 0 Vicryl in a continuous running fashion to secure the mesh to the underlying tissue,

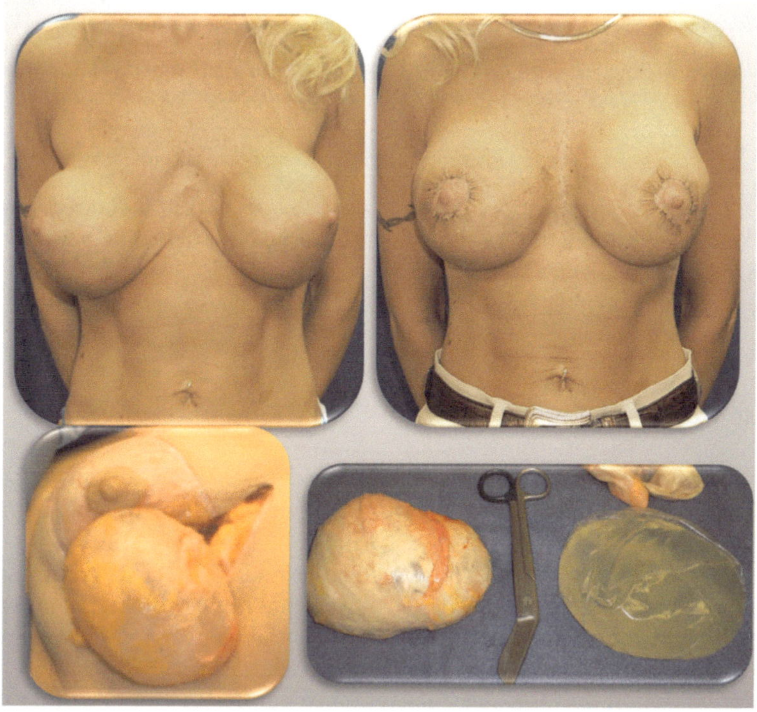

Figure 14.
Grade IV capsular contracture. Patient with grade IV capsular contracture. Patient underwent en bloc capsulectomy with simultaneous breast lift and augmentation.

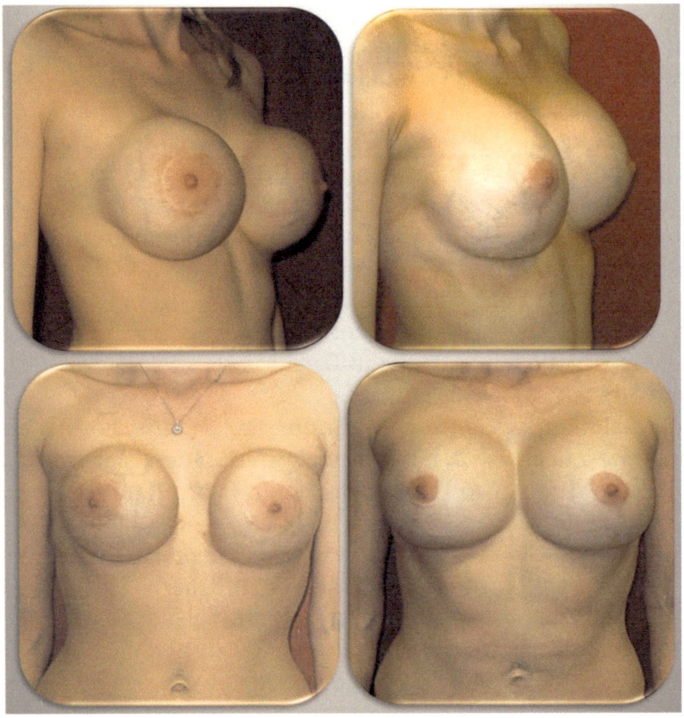

Figure 15.
Recurrent capsular contracture and use of ADM. Patient had developed grade IV capsular contracture following four previous breast augmentation surgeries. Upon evaluation by the authors, residual implant pockets were discovered, in addition to a rolled pectoralis muscle and calcified capsules. The excess scar tissue/capsules were excised, and the pocket was reconstructed with an ADM. The ADM was attached to the inferior edge of the pectoralis muscle and secured to the rib at the desired IMF. A vertical mastopexy was simultaneously performed.

as well as ribs, recreating the internal support. Next, the mesh is fixated to the overlying fascial flap to provide additional soft tissue coverage using a 0 Vicryl (**Figure 15**).

Routine and long-term follow-up is imperative to ensure proper healing and monitor for signs of contracture recurrence.

4.4 Implant rippling/deflation

As previously stated, breast implant rippling occurs when the implant borders fold, resulting in visible wrinkles on the skin. Surgeons must be prepared to offer both minimally invasive and invasive surgical options to address this issue.

Autologous fat grafting can be performed to provide additional volume and soft tissue coverage, particularly in patients with minimal breast thickness. However, there are two main concerns associated with breast fat grafting: variable resorption of the grafted tissue and potential increased cancer risk [28].

Studies have shown that the absorption rate of autologous fat grafting ranges from 20 to 90%, with an average retention of approximately 50% [29, 30]. Complications, such as fat necrosis and oil cyst formation leading to nodules, can occur following grafting. It is important for patients to be informed that around 40–60% of the graft may resorb over a 3–6-month period and that additional grafting sessions may be required to achieve the desired outcome.

Regarding the risk of oncologic transformation, research has indicated that there is no significant increase in tumor recurrence after fat grafting following breast-conserving therapy or mastectomy [31, 32].

During the procedure, fat is harvested from another area of the body and transferred to the breast, enhancing its shape, contour, volume, and thickness. To ensure adequate vascularization, it is recommended to place small amounts of fat along the pectoral and supra-pectoral plane. Surgeons should avoid large-volume grafting to minimize the risk of increased graft pressure, leading to tissue damage and necrosis [33, 34].

Implant exchange is a more invasive option, where the previous implants are removed and replaced by a more cohesive implant. Breast implant cohesiveness is defined as the consistency of the breast implant silicone gel, ranging from low to high cohesiveness. Silicone cohesiveness is determined by the amount of cross-linking of the silicone molecules, providing a stable and solid gel consistency [35]. Selection of the proper implant cohesiveness is based on the patient's desired outcome. High-cohesive implants are ideal for those that desire a more defined and upper pole fullness, while low/moderate cohesive implants provide a more natural feel and adequate shape maintenance. In addition to maintaining the implant shape and fullness, high cohesive implants have a decreased risk of leakage due to their solid-like gel structure.

In cases where implant rippling is due to sub-glandular placement, conversion to a subpectoral plane allows for additional soft tissue. The subpectoral plane allows for additional implant support and reduces the appearance of rippling. A combination of pocket exchange, high implant cohesiveness, and autologous fat grafting may provide an excellent aesthetic result in those patients with minimal soft tissue coverage. While increased cohesiveness offers advantages, such as reduced gel bleed, in the event of rupture, it comes at the expense of implant softness, directly affecting the tactile sensation of the reconstructed or augmented breast [36].

4.5 Complex breast (constricted, asymmetric, and massive ptosis)

Certain breasts are simply challenging from the very start even before any other previous breast surgery. Some of the most common complex issues from a virgin breast involve constricted or tubular breast, severely asymmetric breast, and /or extreme ptosis, such as massive weight loss (MWL) surgery.

Asymmetric breast should not merely be treated with a larger implant on the smaller breast. Our goal is to achieve the most symmetry as possible including both shape, size, and NAC position. To do so typically requires removing the "excess" volume from the larger breast to match the smaller breast while positioning the NAC at the same location on the breast mound. If implants are required, then in most cases the same size implants can be used on both sides after the native breast tissue is made to be the same size. The exception for placing different size or different profile implants often is only for cases where the chest wall (ribs) is very different on one side vs. the other requiring a higher profile implant on the sunken side due to the bony deformity (**Figure 16**).

Constricted or tubular breast can be very challenging and risky. The risk is most notable from a potential increase in vascular compromize after releasing the constricted tissues for expansion or NAC rotation. A "donut" style mastopexy may be

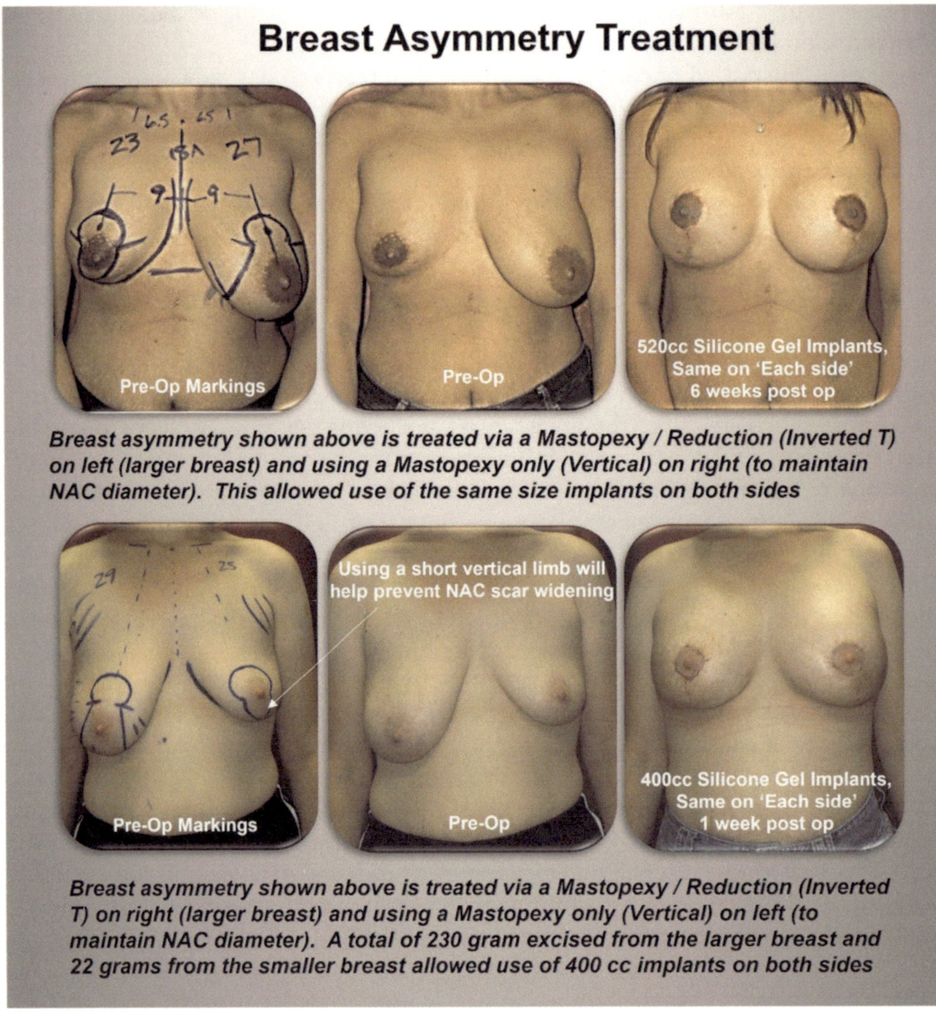

Figure 16.
Asymmetric breast treatment. Treatment of severe breast asymmetry is typically best treated by removing the "excess" tissue from the larger breast as shown in each case above. The same size implants can then be used rather than a much larger implant with very different dimensions on the smaller breast.

beneficial for only small volume tubular breast but has very little benefit for any larger-volume breast. The tissues are often dense and require additional release to get the pedicle to rotate during a vertical or inverted T mastopexy so extra caution must be used to avoid any necrosis. Therefore, large pedunculated and constricted breast should be staged if both a mastopexy and implants are considered (**Figure 17**).

Lastly, extreme ptosis after massive weight loss (MWL) has its own challenges. Due to the poor quality of residual breast tissue, isolated mastopexies are often not enough to give a great and long-lasting result. Often these patients require removal of as much of the excess glandular tissue as possible to lighten the breast, as well as prevent a "waterfall" or "snoopy nose" deformity later when poor quality tissues slide off the implants placed under muscle. So, the goal in MWL breast surgery is frequently to remove as much stretched-out glandular tissue, as well as skin and replace

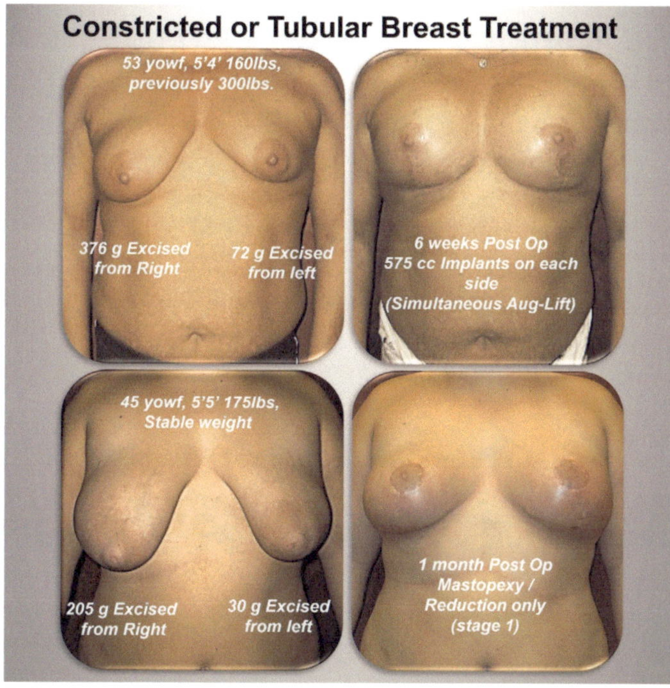

Figure 17.
Constricted or tubular breast treatment. Both patients shown above have "constricted / tubular" type breast with asymmetry. Constriction of the breast can compromize the breast blood supply and increase risk. Both were treated with a superomedial-central pedicle (SMC) mastopexy. However, the patient on top underwent simultaneous breast implant placement with mastopexy. Whereas the patient in the lower picture was treated in 2 stages because her constricted breast was much heavier and carried more risk. Both required excessive tissue to be removed particularly from the larger of the two breasts.

the volume using total submuscular implants. Obviously, if the breast is extremely ptotic or the patient desires extremely large implants then the procedure may require staging (**Figure 18**).

4.6 Nipple-areolar complex refinement/reconstruction

Nipple-areolar complex (NAC) refinement is a crucial component in breast reconstruction. An aesthetically pleasing NAC serves as a cornerstone for achieving an optimal outcome, and it must lie within the surgeon's realm of expertize. Instances warranting NAC refinement span from unsatisfactory outcomes following previous breast reconstruction, NAC asymmetry, disproportionately enlarged NACs, and pronounced discoloration. The goal of refinement is to attain an NAC that embodies naturalness, symmetry, and proportionality.

For patients presenting with NAC irregularities, ranging from minor asymmetries to tubular breasts deformities, a repertoire of mastopexy designs can prove invaluable in restoring the NAC. In cases of minor asymmetries, a crescent lift permits the surgeon to address a vertical discrepancy between the NACs. In cases of tubular breasts with a protruding NAC, a Benelli or Donut mastopexy is beneficial in reducing the projection of the breast mound and concurrently flattening the NAC (**Figure 19**).

After undergoing breast reconstruction, the nipple-areolar complex may lose its proportion and symmetry. An occurrence of NAC widening is particularly common

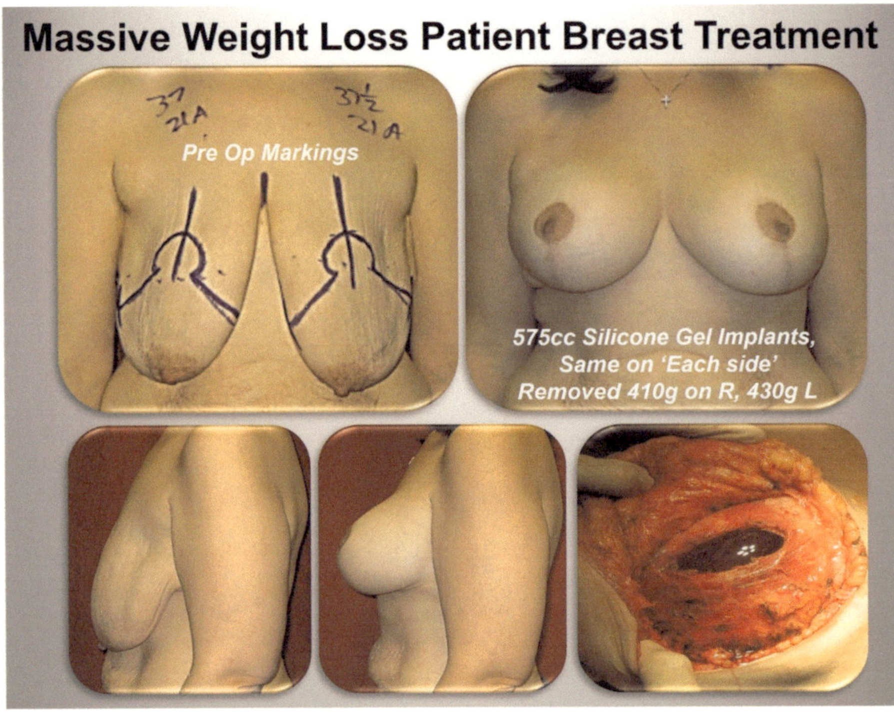

Figure 18.
Severe breast ptosis treatment. Massive weight loss patients like the one shown above who lost 150 lbs., typically require excision of major excess breast tissue and replacement of excised tissue with a total submuscular implant to decrease risk of bottoming out. This will also improve appearance due to the increased implant to tissue ratio (i.e., more implant less natural breast). The key point is that reduction of the poor-quality native breast tissue with help prevent relapse of ptosis and waterfall-type deformity.

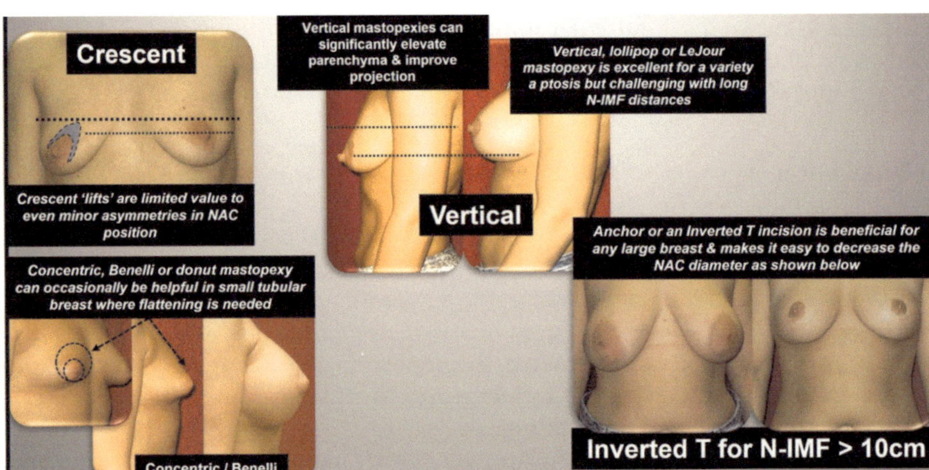

Figure 19.
NAC asymmetry. An array of mastopexy designs may be employed to rectify asymmetries between individual nipple-areolar complexes (NACs) and to harmonize disproportionate NACs.

when a Benelli/donut mastopexy has been performed as this technique can create excess tension along the incision margins. Opting for a vertical mastopexy, either independently or in conjunction with a horizontal component, offers the advantage of

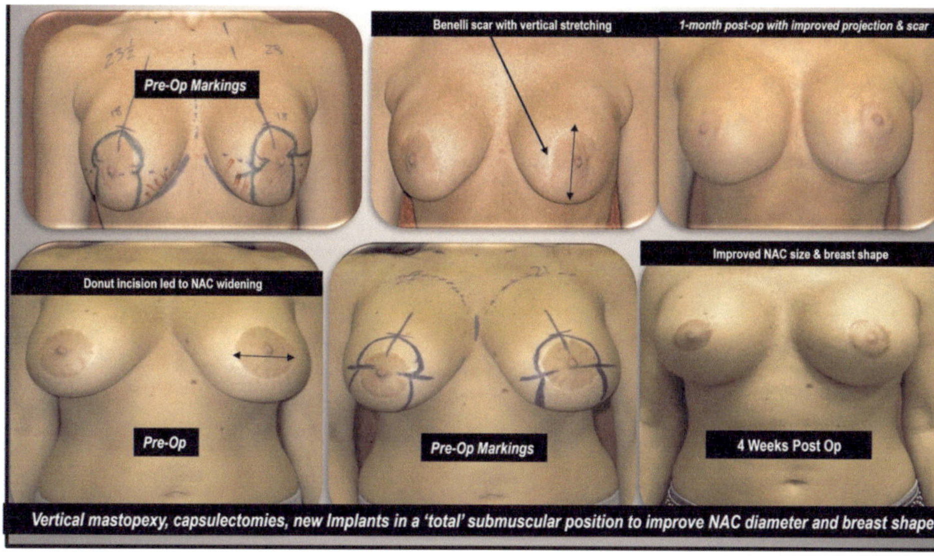

Figure 20.
NAC refinement. The NAC may become disproportionate following breast reconstruction. Performing a vertical mastopexy with or without a horizontal component allows the surgeon to not only address the preexisting scars but also minimize NAC stretching.

distributing tension evenly across the entire incision. This strategic approach not only reduces the risk of NAC widening but also effectively addresses the presence of prior scars (**Figure 20**).

A more recent stride in enhancing breast aesthetics post-reconstruction involves the innovative application of NAC tattooing. Prior breast surgeries can result in NAC distortion, nipple or NAC discoloration, and even nipple necrosis. Proficient tattoo artists possess the ability to emulate the NAC's natural appearance, seamlessly melding it with the adjacent skin. This includes devising a tailored color palette for each patient and artfully imbuing the nipple with texture and dimension, yielding remarkably authentic results.

5. Conclusion

Aesthetic revision breast surgery or surgery for a variety of complex breast issues represents a transformative journey for both the patient and surgeon with the aim to restore the breast form. Through the interplay of meticulous planning, surgical expertize/technique, a deep understanding of each patient's unique needs/desires, and artistic ability, the surgeon is able to recreate beauty while restoring the patient's self-confidence. While the procedure can provide significant benefits, it is essential to consider the potential risks and have realistic expectations about the outcomes. Patients requiring revision breast surgery should research potential surgeons carefully and choose an experienced, surgeon who has a successful track record of performing revisional surgery.

Disclosure statement

The authors have nothing to disclose.

Author details

Angelo Cuzalina[1], Pasquale G. Tolomeo[2]* and Victoria A. Mañón[3]

1 Tulsa Surgical Arts, Tulsa, OK, USA

2 Exquisite Aesthetics, Fall River, MA, USA

3 Bernard and Gloria Katz Department of Oral and Maxillofacial Surgery, UT Health School of Dentistry, Houston, TX, USA

*Address all correspondence to: doctortolomeo@gmail.com

IntechOpen

© 2023 The Author(s). Licensee IntechOpen. This chapter is distributed under the terms of the Creative Commons Attribution License (http://creativecommons.org/licenses/by/3.0), which permits unrestricted use, distribution, and reproduction in any medium, provided the original work is properly cited.

References

[1] ASPA. Plastic Surgery Statistics Report. 2019. Available from: www.plasticsurgery.org/documents/News/Statistics/2019/plastic-surgery-statistics-full-report-2019.pdf

[2] American Cancer Society. American Cancer Society Recommendations for the Early Detection of Breast Cancer. 2022. Available from: https://www.cancer.org/cancer/breast-cancer/screening-tests-and-early-detection/american-cancer-society-recommendations-for-the-early-detection-of-breast-cancer.html

[3] Mallucci P, Branford O. Concepts in aesthetic breast dimensions: Analysis of the ideal breast. Journal of Plastic, Reconstructive & Aesthetic Surgery. 2012;**65**(1):8-16

[4] Janis J. Essentials of Aesthetic Surgery. New York: Thieme; 2017

[5] Stevens W. Grabb and Smith's Plastic Surgery: Mastopexy and Mastopexy/Augmentation. 7th ed. Philadelphia, PA: Wolters Kluwer; 2013

[6] Nahai F, Nahai F. Art of Aesthetic Surgery. 2nd ed. St. Louis, Missouri: Thieme Medical; 2011

[7] Atiye B, Chahine F. Metrics of the aesthetically perfect breast. Aesthetic Plastic Surgery. 2018;**42**(5):1187-1194

[8] Bolletta E, Mcgoldrick C, Hall-Findlay E. Aesthetic breast surgery: What do the measurements reveal? Aesthetic Surgery Journal. 2019;**40**(7):742-752

[9] Bresnick SD. Prophylactic leukotriene inhibitor therapy for the reduction of capsular contracture in primary silicone breast augmentation: Experience with over 1100 cases. Plastic and Reconstructive Surgery. 2017;**139**(2):379-385. DOI: 10.1097/PRS.0000000000003006. Epub: 2017 Jan 26

[10] Headon H, Kasem A, Mokbel K. Capsular contracture after breast augmentation: An update for clinical practice. Archives of Plastic Surgery. 2015;**42**(5):532-543. DOI: 10.5999/aps.2015.42.5.532. Epub: 2015 Sep 15

[11] Frame J. The waterfall effect in breast augmentation. Gland Surgery. 2017;**6**(2):193-202. DOI: 10.21037/gs.2016.10.01

[12] Qureshi A, Myckatyn T, Tenenbaum M. Mastopexy and Mastopexy-augmentation. Aesthetic Surgery Journal. 2018;**38**(4):374-384

[13] Benelli L. A new periareolar mammaplasty: The "round block" technique. Aesthetic Plastic Surgery. 1990;**14**(1):93-100

[14] Cuzalina A, McLain L. Simultaneous Mastopexy with Augmentation. London, UK: IntechOpen; 2019

[15] Hall-Findlay E. Pedicles in vertical breast reduction and mastopexy. Clinics in Plastic Surgery. 2002;**29**(3):379-391

[16] Rohrich R, Gosman A, Brown S, Reisch J. Mastopexy preferences: A survey of board-certified plastic surgeons. Plastic and Reconstructive Surgery. 2006;**118**(7):1631-1638

[17] Siy R, Khan K, Izaddoost S, Brown R. The Superomedial pedicle wise-pattern breast reduction: Reproducible, reliable, and resilient. Seminars in Plastic Surgery. 2015;**29**(02):094-101

[18] Spear SL. Little JW3rd. Breast capsulorrhaphy. Plastic and

Reconstructive Surgery. 1988;**81**(2): 274-279. DOI: 10.1097/00006534-1988 02000-00026

[19] Bradley Calobrace M, Mays C, Wilson R, Wermeling R. Popcorn Capsulorrhaphy in revision aesthetic breast surgery. Aesthetic Surgery Journal. 2020;**40**(1):63-74. DOI: 10.1093/asj/sjy324

[20] Williams SF, Martin DP, Moses AC. The history of GalaFLEX P4HB scaffold. Aesthetic Surgery Journal. 2016;**36** (suppl 2):S33-S42. DOI: 10.1093/asj/ sjw141. Epub: 2016 Oct 3

[21] Narayanan M Nair, Daniel C Mills, Poly-4-Hydroxybutyrate (P4HB) scaffold internal support: Preliminary experience with direct implant opposition during complex breast revisions, Aesthetic Surgery Journal, Volume 39, Issue 11, November 2019, Pages 1203–1213, 10.1093/asj/sjy276

[22] Zeplin PH, Corduff N. Influence of patient age on capsular contracture after aesthetic breast augmentation. The Canadian Journal of Plastic Surgery. 2015;**23**(2):67-69. DOI: 10.1177/ 229255031502300209

[23] Spear SL, Baker JL. Classification of capsular contracture after prosthetic breast reconstruction. Plastic and Reconstructive Surgery. 1995;**96**(5): 1119-1123

[24] Pereira Leite L, Correia Sa I, Marques M. Etiopathogenesis and treatment of breast capsular contracture. Acta Médica Portuguesa. 2013;**26**: 737-745

[25] Lardi AM, Farhadi J. Physiopathology, prevention, and treatment of capsular contracture. In: Urban C et al., editors. Oncoplastic and Reconstructive Breast Surgery. New York: Springer; 2019. pp. 601-607

[26] Moyer HR, Pinell-White X, Losken A. The effect of radiation on acellular dermal matrix and capsule formation in breast reconstruction: Clinical outcomes and histologic analysis. Plastic and Reconstructive Surgery. 2014;**133**(2):214-221. DOI: 10.1097/01.prs.0000437255. 01199.42

[27] Basu CB, Leong M, Hicks MJ. Acellular cadaveric dermis decreases the inflammatory response in capsule formation in reconstructive breast surgery. Plastic and Reconstructive Surgery. 2010;**126**(6):1842-1847. DOI: 10.1097/PRS.0b013e3181f44674

[28] Gutowski KA, ASPS Fat Graft Task Force. Current applications and safety of autologous fat grafts: A report of the ASPS fat graft task force. Plastic and Reconstructive Surgery. 2009;**124**: 272-280

[29] Hivernaud V, Lefourn B, Guicheux J, et al. Autologous fat grafting in the breast: Critical points and technique improvements. Aesthetic Plastic Surgery. 2015;**39**:547-561. DOI: 10.1007/ s00266-015-0503-y

[30] Yin B, Zhang X, Cai L, Han X, Li F. Function-preserving fat grafting in the breast: Results based on 18 years of experience. Journal of Plastic, Reconstructive & Aesthetic Surgery. 2022;**75**(9):2996-3003. DOI: 10.1016/j. bjps.2022.04.084. Epub: 2022 May 2

[31] Petit JY, Botteri E, Lohsiriwat V, et al. Locoregional recurrence risk after lipofilling in breast cancer patients. Annals of Oncology. 2012;**23**:582-588

[32] Kronowitz SJ, Mandujano CC, Liu J, et al. Lipofilling of the breast does not

increase the risk of recurrence of breast cancer: A matched controlled study. Plastic and Reconstructive Surgery. 2016;**137**:385-393

[33] Delay E, Garson S, Tousson G, Sinna R. Fat injection to the breast: Technique, results, and indications based on 880 procedures over 10 years. Aesthetic Surgery Journal. 2009;**29**: 360-376

[34] Khouri RK, Rigotti G, Cardoso E, Khouri RKJ, Biggs TM. Megavolume autologous fat transfer II. Plastic and Reconstructive Surgery. 2014;**133**: 1369-1377

[35] Calobrace MB, Capizzi PJ. The biology and evolution of cohesive gel and shaped implants. Plastic and Reconstructive Surgery. 2014;**134**:6S11S

[36] Handel N, Garcia ME, Wixtrom R. Breast implant rupture: Causes, incidence, clinical impact, and management. Plastic and Reconstructive Surgery. 2013;**132**:11281137